T0074702

MORE
THAN JUST
SURGERY

'So modest is Dr Tehemton Udwadia about his achievements, so willing to accept that he doesn't have all the answers, so open to all forms of healing, that one would never imagine that this is the memoir of a master surgeon of international repute, with a Padma Shri and a Padma Bhushan to boot. In addition, he is a fine writer with an endearing, self-deprecating sense of humour. The book is a delightful memoir, but it is also an important chronicle of empathy in the field of medicine'— Anand Mahindra, chairperson, the Mahindra Group

'*More than Just Surgery* is an action-packed book, with several pearls of wisdom for the budding surgeon, and a liberal sprinkling of fun-filled episodes as the young Udwadia, sometimes in conflict with the powers that be, stands his ground with courage to ultimately gain their respect. Written by a compassionate clinician, a pioneer surgeon-scientist, a dedicated teacher and one with a passion to reach out to rural India to develop the art and science of surgery, this book shows Dr Udwadia as a titan in the field of minimal access surgery. His philosophy has been to challenge the established, restrictive paradigms of waiting for the ideal, and "to do with what you have, both material as well as human resource". In a world driven by profit, Dr Udwadia follows the Gandhian principle of doing more, from less, for more. When the history of access to essential surgical treatment for rural India is eventually written, Dr Udwadia's book will be one of the touchstones that illuminated the path to victory'—Dr Sultan Pradhan, MBBS, MS, FCPS, FRCS (Eng), FACS; president and chief surgical oncologist, Prince Aly Khan Hospital, Mumbai, and consultant surgical oncologist, Breach Candy Hospital and Jaslok Hospital, Mumbai

'Warmth, humility and grace, combined with exceptional skill in specialized surgery, make Dr Tehemton Udwadia a rare commodity. Within these pages resides the story of the making of this truly remarkable human being told in a style that you don't get to see any more. A wonderful account of how values, suffering, hard work, pain and a loving family, along with some absurd and outrageous incidents early in life, have moulded this young Parsee boy into a gem of a person. Hailing from an illustrious family of doctors, Dr Udwadia's service will be long remembered by thousands of people who received his magical touch. If I had to describe him in one phrase, it would be "healer par excellence"'—Harsh Goenka, chairman, RPG Enterprises, and trustee, Breach Candy Hospital Trust

'Tehemton Udwadia is considered, internationally, the father of laparoscopy in India. While the majority of surgical leaders remained sceptical, those with vision and imagination saw the possibilities, and transformed surgery. The very special pioneers shared two additional traits, a desire to educate all surgeons who wanted to learn, and a desire to safely apply the opportunity to all who might benefit, rich or poor. Tehemton Udwadia is that kind of leader. His contributions have been recognized with honorary membership to many of the world's most honorific surgical organizations'—John G. Hunter, MD, FACS, FRCS; professor of surgery, executive vice president and CEO, Oregon Health and Science University, Portland, US

'I have thoroughly enjoyed reading all the chapters. The memoir reflects Dr Udwadia's incredible qualities as a human being and a renowned world-leading surgeon, who is a dear friend to me. The international surgical community would love to read this book'—Prof. Sir Alfred Cuschieri, MD, PhD, ChM, DSc, FRSE, FRCS (Eng), FRCS (Ed), FACS (Hon), FMedSci, RSB; emeritus professor of surgery, molecular oncology and surgical technology, University of Dundee, and emeritus professor to several prestigious universities and colleges

'Very few doctors have the knack of writing a book on medicine that can be easily understood by the layman. Even fewer surgeons have that ability. Dr Tehemton Udwadia is one of those rare few. *More than Just Surgery* is a beautifully written memoir, laced with humour and oozing with compassion. Tehemton has a light touch, and the empathy so needed between surgeon and patient shines through'— Rahul Singh, former editor, *Reader's Digest, Indian Express, Sunday Observer* and *Khaleej Times*, and convener of the Khushwant Singh Literary Festival, and columnist and writer

'Tehemton Udwadia has written this book straight from the heart—not a whiff of a ghost writer. It is an engaging, humorous and often touching read. Even for those of us who have never wielded a scalpel, it is, for the most part, easy to understand and enjoy. And in the midst of all the surgical melodrama and personal snippets, there are some invaluable lessons that he has learnt, and passes on to the reader. Despite his sixty-plus years as a brilliant surgeon, I wonder if he would consider a change in profession'—Dorab R. Sopariwala, political commentator and editorial adviser to NDTV

'Tehemton Udwadia lays down his scalpel to pick up a pen and tell of his unputdownable life. *More than Just Surgery* is a work of grace and gratitude to his mentor, Dr Erach Udwadia, his father, who treated the neediest in Bombay for sixty-four years. The book recounts good deeds and good thoughts, to which Udwadia now adds good words with a Zoroastrian flourish'—Gerson da Cunha, actor, social activist and author

'This book is a treat and I believe it will serve as an inspiration for doctors. Apart from Dr Udwadia's sincerity and commitment to his patients, what stands out is his humility. Of special interest to me is the chapter dedicated to his father, who taught him many valuable lessons. Dr Udwadia is a hidden saint, in secret communion with god, quietly making a difference wherever he goes'—Dr Sudhansu Bhattacharyya, MBBS, MS (General Surgery), MS (Thoracic Surgery), FIACS (India); ex professor of cardiovascular surgery, Seth G.S. Medical College and KEM Hospital, and consultant cardiovascular surgeon, Breach Candy Hospital and several tertiary care hospitals, Mumbai

MORE THAN JUST SURGERY

LIFE LESSONS BEYOND THE O.T.

DR TEHEMTON ERACH UDWADIA

EBURY
PRESS

An imprint of Penguin Random House

EBURY PRESS

USA | Canada | UK | Ireland | Australia
New Zealand | India | South Africa | China

Ebury Press is part of the Penguin Random House group of companies
whose addresses can be found at global.penguinrandomhouse.com

Published by Penguin Random House India Pvt. Ltd
4th Floor, Capital Tower 1, MG Road,
Gurugram 122 002, Haryana, India

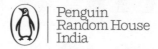

Penguin
Random House
India

First published in Ebury Press by Penguin Random House India 2021

ISBN 9780670096510

Typeset in Minion Pro by Manipal Technologies Limited, Manipal
Printed at Thomson Press India Ltd, New Delhi

www.penguin.co.in

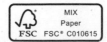

MIX
Paper
FSC FSC® C010615

For
Khorshed
Rushad, Dinaz and Ashad

Contents

Preface

My first brush with medicine was at the clinic of my father, who, for sixty-four years, worked as a general practitioner (GP) in the poorest part of Mumbai (then Bombay)—the mill districts of Lower Parel. I saw how he dedicated his life to healing the sick and how deeply he cared for them.

From 1951, when I was a medical student to the present day, I have not only witnessed first-hand the avalanche of surgical progress, but also seen lives being saved as a result of these advances, be it the disposable plastic syringe or a liver transplant. The past seventy-odd years have also taught me that it is not merely operating skills that make a good surgeon. The purpose of *More than Just Surgery* is not just to chronicle my journey as I grew from a student through residency, research, surgical practice and surgical teaching but also to highlight the lessons it has taught me.

Throughout this period, my journey has been very fortuitously enhanced by a series of 'accidents' that created an exciting albeit tortuous path over a terrain I had neither the intent nor the talent to traverse. My colleagues and peers kindly attribute a great deal to my 'talent', unaware that unexpected and often inexplicable circumstances have placed me in a position from where I have been propelled forward.

The past decades have seen the stupendous growth of Indian surgery. I am convinced that surgery here, across all our tertiary care and most of our teaching hospitals, is comparable to the best in the world. Having said that, my proximity to rural surgery—despite being a city surgeon—gives me a far more complete picture of the trials and tribulations of surgery in India. It is to drive home this point that I participated actively in international surgical societies and their events—to showcase the merit of our urban surgery capabilities, the calibre and strength of our small town and rural surgery, the sad lack of surgical care in remote rural India and, hopefully, to motivate the rich and over-provided to help all developing countries.

Sadly, over the last seventy years, I have realized that for this fantastic progress, we have had to pay a very heavy price. When I started surgery, the surgeon could do no wrong. The bond the patient shared with the surgeon was so strong that the surgeon was looked upon as part of the patient's family. The picture is totally different today. The patient often views the surgeon with mistrust and apprehension, even fear. And not always without reason. If we have any hope of restoring the relationship of complete trust that existed earlier, we should return to talking with, listening to, and touching and feeling the patient with sincere empathy and concern, regardless of their socio-economic background.

I am appalled at how fast the memory of my mentors, as also that of my colleagues, is fading—that generation of surgeons laid the foundation of Indian surgery. If we forget our roots, we have no heritage. Some mentors are mentioned in the pages of this book. Many more, equally revered, are not. Within these pages, I also wanted to acknowledge the contributions that have been made by my colleagues, peers, residents, students and nurses. And, most importantly, what I have learnt from every single patient.

More than Just Surgery aims to be a warm, personal account of people, incidents, mentors, failures and absurdities set against the backdrop of surgery—a historical recounting through the eyes and hands of someone who has lived through the journey.

Mumbai, 2021   Tehemton Erach Udwadia

1

My First Surgery

I woke up with a start. There was heavy pounding on my door. I was momentarily disoriented but then it registered. I was asleep in my room at the residents' quarters of the Bai Jerbai Wadia Hospital for Children, Bombay (now Mumbai). It was about 3 a.m. on the first day of my first job as a house surgeon on 1 January 1957. While checking into the hospital the previous evening, the receptionist handed me the keys to my room and informed me that all surgical residents had taken leave for New Year's Eve. I was the locum—temporary replacement—for their calls. The pounding grew louder. I was needed immediately in the operating theatre (OT).

I was a bundle of nerves as I approached the theatre. When I opened the door, in my panicked condition, the OT appeared as large as a badminton hall with huge windows on two sides and a wall across from the door. A light was hanging from the high ceiling over the operation table. There was a pool of blood on the floor. A boy, who looked about ten years of age, was lying quietly on the operation table while a nurse sat beside him and stroked his head. A theatre assistant was suctioning blood from the boy's mouth. I was ashamed to note that the child was far more relaxed than I was.

Gingerly walking around the blood, I approached the table. As soon as the nurse saw me, she said crisply, 'Good morning, doctor. Happy New Year. Please come in.' She added, 'I am Sister Alvares, the theatre superintendent. I have been here for four years. This is Laxman, the theatre assistant, and he has been here for thirty years. I am sorry there is no one else to assist us as I have sent all my junior girls away for New Year's Eve. This child is bleeding from the tonsil fossa after a tonsillectomy done six days ago.' (The tonsils lie in a fossa or a cavity on both sides of the mouth behind the last molar tooth.) I envied her calm. I, on the other hand, was looking down the barrel of my first surgical procedure and struggling to maintain my composure.

She covered the child's face with a cloth mask and started spraying ethyl chloride on the mask. When the boy was quiet, she started dribbling ether on it. This was the standard protocol for inducing anaesthesia in the 1950s—start with ethyl chloride and continue with ether. The ether was poured drop by drop in a circular manner. As a student, I was told that it was called the *jalebi* method of administering anaesthesia. It may seem primitive but, in fact, it required greater skill than today's sophisticated procedures. It also required total awareness of the patient, especially when children were involved. There was no monitoring equipment—all we had then to judge oxygenation levels were the patient's pulse, blood pressure and nail colour!

As soon as the boy was anaesthetized, Sister called me to the head of the table. She removed the ether mask, placed a curved red rubber tube in my hand and said that we needed to intubate the patient. I had seen—but never carried out—an intubation. Sister could sense my nervousness. Intubation is the procedure in which a tube is inserted into the windpipe so that anaesthetic gases can be provided directly to the lungs.

Sister first inserted a laryngoscope—an instrument with a light at its tip—to illuminate the vocal cords. Then, she held my hand that was holding the red tube and gently guided it between the vocal cords into the windpipe. The boy was now intubated. Deftly removing the laryngoscope, she fixed the rubber tube to the boy's right cheek with adhesive tape and quickly attached it to the anaesthesia machine so that the ether and oxygen could go continuously into the boy's lungs at a controlled rate. Laxman, who was holding the boy while he was being anaesthetized, moved to the head of the table and started checking the flow of ether and the child's pulse.

Sister and I quickly scrubbed, gowned and gloved. I was now standing on the right side of the patient, Sister was on his left, and Laxman at his head. Using a tongue spatula, Sister made sure the boy's mouth was wide open. Laxman repositioned the top light exactly on to the bleeding fossa. To arrest the bleeding, I had to suture the pillars, Sister told me. When the tonsils are removed, the fossa is what you can see between the two tissue folds or pillars. The bleeding was from the left fossa.

Sister gave me a peculiar harpoon-like bent needle with a thread in its eye. I'd never seen such a needle before. Again, holding my hand, she gently rotated her wrist so that the needle pierced through both the pillars. She then reversed the wrist movement and took the needle out, leaving the thread in the boy's mouth. 'Please tie a knot,' she said.

One of the things I'd enjoyed most as a medical student was to suture skin in the casualty department. I was good at tying surgical knots but here, I had to tie a knot deep in a young child's throat—something I'd never done before. Sister whispered in my ear, 'Tie a surgeon's knot.' The surgeon's knot is where you have a double throw of the first knot, so that it does not slip and get loose before the second knot is tied. To my great surprise, I managed to tie the knot deep in the fossa. Sister then cut the thread short, rethreaded the needle and handed it to me. This time, as the needle tip was about to be put through the pillar, Sister left me to do it on my own. I imitated the way Sister had rotated her wrist and carefully took the second stitch through both the pillars. I then withdrew the needle exactly as she had done, making sure that the thread was still in the child's mouth. With a nod of approval, she said, 'Tie the knot exactly as you did earlier.' I did so again, this time more deftly. The bleeding reduced to a trickle.

'Very good, doctor. *You* stopped the bleeding,' Sister told me with a smile, with the emphasis on *you*. At first, I thought she was being sarcastic, but then realized that her tone was genuine—one of confidence and support. As we observed the boy, I suddenly started feeling faint. My legs began to wobble. The OT now had another patient—me. Realizing I was about to fall, Laxman rushed to my side, held both my arms and lowered me gently on to a stool. I felt nauseous; my mouth was dry, and I was dripping with sweat.

Meanwhile, Sister was gently pressing a piece of gauze on the child's tonsil fossa. After ten minutes, she confirmed that the bleeding had completely stopped and removed the red tube from the windpipe. As the child started coming out of the anaesthesia, she turned him on his side. Both child and surgeon recovered slowly together, while Laxman produced cups of hot coffee for Sister and me.

As a student, I had not just seen consultants and registrars, but even house surgeons and students talk down to nurses. Even if it was not with disdain, it certainly wasn't with respect. I realized that this nurse had done the entire procedure while holding my hand but had given me credit for it. She had done it gently, encouragingly and expertly. I was full of gratitude, respect and admiration for this nurse who I had never seen before. From her, I learnt the lesson that if you are helping someone, you should do so with grace. I was also amazed that a ward boy or a theatre assistant could work as an anaesthetist and look after both the patient and a panic-stricken surgeon. You don't learn just from surgeons or senior surgical residents. The very first mentors in my surgical career were a nurse and a theatre assistant.

After penning this episode, I read it again and was amazed at how I could recall the minute details of my very first experience as a surgeon that had taken place sixty-four years ago. While most other operations I have done are a bit of a blur, this one will always remain fresh in my mind. The fact that I saw blood on the floor when I entered the theatre, and consciously made sure I did not step on it. How the nurse saw the panic on my face and reassured both patient and doctor at the same time. These memories will remain with me till the end of my days.

After we finished our coffee, Sister said that we could shift the child to the ward. I got up from the stool, but since my legs were still unsteady, Laxman walked with me to my room.

I went to bed with my clothes on. Laxman turned off the lights and left.

That night, sleep was hard to come by. I went down for rounds later in the morning, especially to see the child who I had performed surgery on. His parents were near the bed and his mother had tears in her eyes. She and the father thanked me for saving their son. I was very embarrassed and did not know what to say as the truth was that I was clueless throughout the procedure. It had, in effect, been done by Sister Alvares.

And that is how New Year's Day started for me in 1957.

2

Growing Up in Bombay

I think the best thing to do when writing an account of one's journey in surgery is to start from the place where it all began. For me, that was Banoo Manor, my first real memory. As I look back on my eighty-seven-odd years, my first clear memory is of my parents, my elder brother Farokh and I, moving to a house called Banoo Manor near Bombay's Chowpatty Beach. I was five. It was 1939, just before the Second World War.

Bombay then was a very different city from the one that we know today as Mumbai. It was much cleaner, had fewer people, far fewer cars and no taxis. Transportation was by train (we had two tracks of electric trains even then), bus, tram or Victoria—horse-drawn carriages named after the

British Queen. Mornings started at 6 with the milkman, the newspaper man and the *baidawala*, and were a crazy rush: get dressed, check homework, gulp down a breakfast of milk, egg, bread and delicious Polson butter and rush to catch the school bus before Maka, the driver, drove off. During the day, there was tranquillity till the children returned home from school and came out to play cricket in the open spaces. Shouts of 'out' or 'run out' were sometimes punctuated by the shattering of a neighbour's window by a cricket ball. Everyone would be back home by 7 p.m. We'd do our homework ourselves, read books, listen to the radio, make models or write to pen pals all over the world. Evenings would usually be so quiet that one could often hear the patter of the barefoot lamplighters running around with their long poles to light the street's gas lamps. Sundays were family days, spent visiting grandparents, uncles, cousins or catching the occasional movie. No gadgets, no gimmicks.

On Sundays, the police or naval bands would perform at the Chowpatty Bandstand to packed audiences. On some evenings, we would go to the famous Naaz Restaurant on top of Malabar Hill for falooda and samosas. The view from there was breathtaking—a wide blue bay; clean, shimmering sand; the imposing steeple of Afghan Church, the Colaba lighthouse, ships in the harbour, small islands in the distance—all bathed in the red glow of the setting sun.

Banoo Manor, named after my grandmother, had been built by my grandfather. Our apartment on the ground floor had four large bedrooms, a huge sitting and dining room, and a kitchen, but only one bathroom and one toilet, Indian-style. Cooking was done on a coal fire. My father was a doctor, a GP. He had two dispensaries in the Lower Parel and Dongri areas of the city, but also treated patients at home—one of the bedrooms served as a dispensary. Daddy worked very hard and would be exhausted and sweaty when he returned home at night. When I was young, I thought he was very rich because he would come back with lots of coins. Only much later did I realize that he didn't get currency notes because he worked in a very poor part of town. On returning home, Daddy would take off his jacket—he always wore a tie and jacket to work—and put it on one of the handles of the two Godrej cupboards in his bedroom. On the other handle was Daddy's second jacket; he wore his jackets on alternate days. All our clothes were made of cotton and stitched by a tailor who came once a year to our house to take our measurements. If Farokh's old clothes fit me, I didn't get new ones. Unlike Farokh, I was mischievous and would often get a scolding and occasionally a beating. If it hurt too much, I would go quietly to Daddy's bedroom, and smell the armpit of his coat. That soothed and comforted me.

Within a year of moving to Banoo Manor, my parents had another son. Named Darius, he was also called the 'War Child' since he'd been born after the war had started. Mummy was a strict disciplinarian who insisted on us boys keeping fixed hours for everything. During the war, Mummy was in the navy and used to wear a very smart uniform. Her section was staffed entirely with women who worked on coding and decoding highly classified messages of allied and enemy ship movements. Mummy used to joke that she reported to Lord Mountbatten. But for us, the biggest advantage of her job was that she could use the military canteen and get us Kraft cheese and condensed milk tins. She was also an excellent pianist. Next to our house was the Barrister Gymkhana with its vast grounds and three tennis courts, which had been converted into a camp for English soldiers. Mummy would play the piano every evening with the doors of the living room wide open. Soldiers would gather on the other side of the barbed wire fence to listen. When she played wartime songs like 'My Bonnie Lies Over the Ocean' and 'White Cliffs of Dover', the soldiers would sing along. But when it was my turn to play the piano, they'd all go away.

As soon as he came back from work, Daddy would turn on our small black radio and listen to the BBC. He used to get very upset at setbacks to the Allied forces and would animatedly discuss the news over the telephone with his friends. Our telephone was very old-fashioned and had two parts—one was the base, which was nothing but a vertical stand with a circular ring at the bottom with numbers for dialling and the mouthpiece on the top; the other was the earpiece which hung on a hook attached to the vertical stand.

During the war years, rice, wheat, sugar, kerosene and petrol were rationed. While doctors were entitled to more fuel than other car owners, Daddy's quota wasn't enough for him to be able to drive to his dispensaries and back home. So he had to go part of the way by train. Luckily, vegetables, mutton and fish were not rationed. Neither was chicken but, in those days, chicken was very expensive. Twice a week, Daddy would go to Chowpatty Bazaar, down the lane from our house, for provisions. Very often, I would go with him. I liked that—I was always happy to have an excuse not to study.

When patients came by our house early in the morning to be examined by my father before he left for work, they would often take back mixtures made by him, and I would try to help. By the time I was twelve, Daddy had taught me to make basic medicines like 'Mixt Soda Sal' which was the standard preparation for fever, aches and pains. There were very few pharmaceutical companies in those times and almost all of them were foreign. They wouldn't give the doctor gifts such as the pens and other merchandise you see today but booklets of information. The first page of one Glaxo booklet had only one sentence, 'The hand of the Chirurgeon is the hand of God.' Chirurgeon, Daddy told me, was French for surgeon. Why wasn't he a surgeon, I asked. He replied that he'd been a house surgeon for one-and-a-half years after his MBBS, but then had to stop to earn money to support his parents. His mother was ill, his father had retired without a pension, his eldest brother was in China and his other brother was disabled and couldn't work. So, Daddy started working as a GP. Did he still want to be a surgeon, I asked. He said he was very content in general practice but would be happy if one of his sons became a surgeon. That stayed with me.

Mummy was always very concerned about our education. Initially, she had put both Farokh and me in the Senior Cambridge section of St Mary's, a very good school. But when she learnt that students in the Matriculation section could go to college after passing their eighth standard whereas students in the Senior Cambridge section had to wait until they passed their ninth, she immediately had us transferred. I preferred the Matric section. Unlike Cambridge, these children came from all walks of life—from the very rich to the very poor—and their education was subsidized by the school. Mummy would come to St Mary's regularly by tram to discuss me with the principal, Father Molina. She was not worried about Farokh since he was a good student. But because I was mischievous and not studious, she used to enquire about me. Luckily, Father had a soft spot for me—he'd tell her that I was his best student and that she shouldn't worry. That made me feel very special and close to him.

One day, in 1944, as Farokh and I were returning home by school bus, we heard a deafening noise. The bus shook, and we thought Bombay was being bombed. Later, we learnt that the ammunition on a ship in the dock had accidentally caught fire and exploded. Many people were killed and injured and the entire dock area was on fire.

After the war was over, all the students were very happy that the Allies had won and celebrated as though it was their own victory. The independence movement was strong even among the student community. I remember that on one occasion, in 1946, when the Governor of Bombay Presidency—I think his name was Colville—was passing by St Mary's School in his car, all the students gathered near the gate and shouted 'Inquilab Zindabad'. I was thirteen when India became independent and, with Daddy holding my hand tightly, went to Chowpatty Beach to listen to a speech by Mahatma Gandhi. There was a huge crowd but it was all very orderly.

School wasn't only about studies. When I was in the seventh grade, I represented St Mary's in the Harris Shield Interschool Cricket Tournament and we made it to the third round. After the holidays, we found to our dismay, especially mine, that Father Molina had been called back to Spain and an Indian priest had been made principal. The two men could not have been more different: whereas Father Molina was a kind, forgiving man, the new principal was a harsh disciplinarian. I couldn't get along with him.

He would constantly pick on me, though I must admit that I was not entirely blameless.

Although we'd done reasonably well in the Harris cricket tournament, the new principal said he wasn't going to pay the fees for the next year since he thought 'there was no chance we'd win'. We were all outraged. We told the other teachers what the principal had said and added that we were ready to raise the money ourselves. The teachers promised to speak to the principal. Meanwhile, during a free period one day, I stood on my desk and gave a passionate speech saying that we had to tell the Jesuits in Spain to immediately send Father Molina back. The new principal had no business being in the school, I declared. There was wild cheering as I spoke, and then sudden pin-drop silence. I turned around to find the principal standing behind me. Summoning me to his office, he suspended me from school.

With a strict mother like mine, you could imagine what was going through my mind. Fortunately, Mummy had gone to visit her grandmother in Pune (then Poona). I told Daddy that I had been given special leave to stay at home and study for the SSC exams. Daddy, gentle soul that he was, believed me. But as soon as my mother came back, she realized something was amiss. She met the principal and was told that I could not be permitted to take the exams as a St Mary's boy; I would have to appear as an ex-student.

1949 was the first year of the SSC examinations, which replaced the matriculation exam. When I got my results, I had very good marks. I immediately got admission into Wilson College. It was a family tradition—my father went to Wilson, Farokh had passed his Inter Science through Wilson and now, it was my turn. I had hardly been in college for a week when the names of candidates who stood first in various subjects in the SSC examination were announced in the newspapers. To my surprise, I had stood first in English from Bombay Presidency. At that time, the presidency included what is now Maharashtra, a part of Karnataka, a part of Madhya Pradesh and most of Gujarat. All my teachers called to congratulate me. But my success created a dilemma for the school. The SSC board gave scholarships to those who stood first in a subject—but they had to be students of a recognized school. Since I had appeared as an ex-student, I didn't qualify, unless I was reinstated. So, the principal had no choice but to readmit me. To my great joy, he was forced to tell the entire school, masters included, at the daily assembly and in my presence, that I was a good sportsman and a model student who had brought honour to the school!

On joining Wilson College, I enrolled in the National Cadet Corps (NCC). I loved it. We had a parade twice a week on the college campus, and I made sure that my uniform was well-ironed; and my heavy military boots and belt buckle were polished to a high gloss. Tough Second World War veterans from the Grenadiers and Dogra regiments put us through our paces. They would regale us with thrilling stories of the battles they'd fought. Professor Wagh, head of the Mathematics department, was my platoon commander and the two of us got along very well. I still remember a three-week NCC camp in Deolali that we had gone to in December 1949. We slept in open barracks even though it was bitterly cold, had to get up at 5 a.m. and struggle with frozen fingers to lace up our boots. I strongly believe that the NCC is a great way of bringing together youngsters from different parts of the country so that they develop discipline and an all-India spirit. Around this time, my mother gave birth to my third sibling and her fourth son, Firdaus, who was fourteen years younger than me.

Meanwhile, as my first-year college exams approached, I grew increasingly worried. At that time, two years of college were required before you could study law, medicine or engineering. The first year was followed by the Inter or second year. I was hopeless at arithmetic and since we had to pass in all subjects, I was afraid I'd fail and not make it to Inter. (In fact, I'd only done so well in the SSC because arithmetic was not in the mathematics curriculum and I had no problems with algebra and geometry.) I was so desperate that I wrote a letter to Prof. Wagh on my arithmetic exam answer sheet requesting him to pass me. I said that I'd enjoyed being in his NCC platoon and pointed out that since I planned to become a doctor, I didn't really need to know much arithmetic.

That letter proved to be a godsend. Prof. Wagh, to his eternal credit, awarded me thirty-five marks, the bare minimum required to pass! Now, forever free of arithmetic, I studied as hard as I could, since my performance in the Inter exams would determine whether I'd get admission into medical college. Farokh had got a first class in his Inter, but I knew that I'd never be able to match his grades. So, I prepared a back-up plan. I'd do my damnedest best to become at least a sergeant in the NCC, get a BSc degree and join the Indian Air Force as a pilot.

The Inter Science exams had both theory and practicals. My theory exam went reasonably well, and I thought I'd get about 50 per cent. But the minimum overall range needed to get into medical college was 58 to 60 per cent. After the theory exam came the practicals. The first was biology which, fortunately, was held at Wilson College. We had to appear for both zoology and botany practicals. In botany, I had no problem with the exam because I had a section of the stem stained perfectly. But in zoology, I had a cockroach for dissection and made a hash of it by badly mutilating it. Time was ticking away and I didn't know what to do. With twenty minutes left for the bell, a Wilson College lecturer walked by, picked up the mangled cockroach from my table, put it in his pocket and replaced it with a juicy new one. This time I made no mistake—I finished dissecting the insect to perfection just as the bell rang.

The chemistry practicals, my weak link, were held at St Xavier's College. The laboratory was so large and there were so many shelves with so many bottles full of chemicals in front of me that I knew that just locating the ones I needed for my experiments was going to be a problem. On my left was a tall boy and to my right a short girl with glasses. When I smiled at the boy, he turned his face away. I then turned to the girl. She smiled back. I gathered my courage and placed the slip of paper on which the experiment I had to perform was written close to her table, so she could read it too. I then asked where the sulphuric acid bottle that I needed for my experiment was. She said I needed hydrochloric acid, not sulphuric acid, and pointed to the right bottle. And so, with her often showing me the right reagent to use, I finished my practicals.

I expected an overall percentage of about 50. But when the results were announced, I was over the moon. I'd got about 44 per cent in my theory but 75 per cent in my practicals. Put together, that was more than enough. I was admitted to the 1951 batch of Bombay's GS Medical College and KEM Hospital. Had it not been for those kind souls seventy years ago, I wonder where I would have ended up. By the happy accident of a benevolent mathematics professor, a replaced cockroach and help from a remarkable female student, I was to become a surgeon.

3

Medical School

Bombay's second and India's twelfth medical teaching facility, Seth Gordhandas Sunderdas (GS) Medical College was founded by the heirs of Seth Gordhandas Sunderdas, a wealthy cloth merchant. After his death, they agreed to fund a medical school on the condition that all the professors and students at the institute would be Indian, in response to Grant Medical College's mandate that all its teachers be English. It opened in 1925 with forty-six students. The college was attached to King Edward Memorial (KEM) Hospital, run by the municipality for the poor in the city. The institutions were connected by corridors so that students, doctors and patients could easily move between the two. Bombay's top surgeons and physicians treated patients and taught students from 9 a.m. to 1 p.m. for no remuneration, which was the norm for decades in several teaching hospitals and was considered to be a privilege. There would be dozens of applications for one post and only the best would be selected.

In the first week of June 1951, eighty young men and women, of which I was one, entered GS Medical College on the first day of the term. The dean, Dr Dhayagude, addressed us. He said we needed to be committed, studious, honest and compassionate doctors. We had five years of studying ahead of us. Our first two years, he went on, would consist of lectures in anatomy, physiology and biochemistry for the first MBBS exam. Pharmacology would be added for the second MBBS exam and we'd be tested in seven subjects during the final MBBS exam.

We were taken around the college and were very impressed by the imposing statue of Dr Shirvalkar, a former honorary professor of surgery, in the main foyer. The high ceilings, wide staircases and big lecture halls whose seating was so well designed that a student on the last bench could get as good a view of the teacher as a student on the first, were all equally striking. We also got a glimpse of the canteen, lunchroom, badminton hall, three tennis courts and men's and ladies' hostels spread across the generously proportioned campus.

However, we were in for a shock the following day when we entered the vast anatomy dissection hall. On the tables were treated corpses, the dead bodies. The hall reeked of formalin, a chemical used to preserve cadavers. In the 1950s, this and other preservatives were injected into the blood vessels immediately after death so that the corpse would not decompose and remain in the normal anatomical state, even though they were somewhat shrunken and mummified. Formalin gave off an odour which was unpleasant, pungent and distinctive. It went into our noses, got into our clothes and our eyes, and identified us as first-year students as it followed us wherever we went during the first few weeks.

All of us had to purchase Cunningham's *Manual of Practical Anatomy*. This legendary three-volume text—copies of which I still have—was our Bible. It described every organ, vessel, nerve, muscle and bone in the body. In addition to this text, each batch had to have a set of dissection instruments. Dr Desai, the head anatomy demonstrator, told us that we would be divided into batches of four and each batch would be given one body part to dissect. We'd begin with the superior extremities (arms) and inferior extremities (legs) as they were the least complex parts of the body. The abdomen, thorax, neck, head, face and brain were reserved for later.

My friend from Wilson College, Raja Dhurandar, with whom I used to play tennis regularly, had also joined GS and we decided to combine forces. As we were talking, a tall, distinguished-looking boy came up and asked if he could join us. We both agreed. His name was Edmond D'Souza and he was from Singapore. He was five years older than us because the Japanese had occupied Singapore during the Second World War and all academic activities had come to a standstill. The fourth member of our group was Atul Lakhia, a very quiet and intense fellow.

Unlike the other three in my group and most of the other students in the batch, I found dissection fascinating and totally absorbing. I'd decided to become a surgeon and felt that the best way to start was to dissect as much as I could. Raja didn't like to use his hands; he wanted to be a physician anyway. I ended up doing most of the dissecting, with Edmond reading the text from Cunningham's manual very clearly. Raja and Atul would nod their heads in confirmation if I was showing the correct structure. We didn't wear gloves and the formalin wrinkled the skin on my fingers and hands. Today, due to the paucity of bodies and limited space, anatomy is taught using computers, virtual reality and 3D printing. But I remain convinced that dissecting a body from head to toe is the best way to learn anatomy.

Both our physiology teachers—Dr Batliwala, who was the head of physiology, and Dr Monteiro, the assistant professor—were very good. But I found physiology practicals somewhat disagreeable. Almost invariably, we used a frog. We had to first 'pith' it—i.e., put a sharp, long instrument into its spinal cord to paralyse it below the neck. It didn't feel any pain but I found pithing inhumane and always got someone else to do it. I have to admit, though, that these practicals enabled us to thoroughly study the frog's muscle and cardiac activity, its nerve function and dysfunction, and so on. Physiology also involved histology—studying the microscopic structure of various tissues and organs and using different stains to make the tissue parts and organs stand out.

These days, senior students 'rag' new entrants, sometimes even physically harming them. But that's not how things were in 1951. In fact, the second-year students threw a party for us in the main lecture hall with the dean in attendance. They gave speeches saying how happy they were that we'd joined the college and how they were ready to help us whenever necessary. I replied on our batch's behalf—it was the first time I'd spoken into a microphone. We then went to the badminton hall where snacks had been laid out. Games had been organized for the two batches to play together and get to know each other better.

Among that batch of second-year students were two boys with whom I've fortunately had a lot to do throughout my career— Praful Desai and G.B. Parulkar. It was a very happy evening.

I also used to go regularly for cricket practice—at the grounds of Grant Medical College next to Wilson College Gymkhana during my first two years, and then, for the next three at GS's new sports complex, named after the famous gynaecologist Dr B.N. Purandare. We'd have matches every weekend—half day on Saturdays and full days on Sundays. I played for GS in the Intercollegiate Cricket Tournament all through my five years of MBBS and, in my final year, I was voted captain. At the Annual Athletics competitions, I also won the discus throw event, and the 100- and 200-metre sprints. Our batch won the relays over both these distances. Every year, we had a three-day break during which we had music recitals, plays, dances and a one-day picnic. We would go home exhausted, hoarse after shouting our battle cry, 'GSMC, GSMC ALWAYS AT THE TOP, GSMC, GSMC, OUR WINNING WAYS NEVER STOP!'

At the first MBBS exam after our first two years, I was expecting a distinction in anatomy and reasonable marks in physiology. That was not to be. I got a distinction in physiology. But, in the anatomy practicals, I had a sudden moment of amnesia and wrongly identified the chordae tendineae, one of the structures in the heart, as the choroid plexus, a structure in the brain. It was a major mistake. I was failed. But when I took the exam again, I passed with distinction.

After the first MBBS exam, our hospital training at KEM began. My first surgical posting was under Professor P.K. Sen, a brilliant and pioneering surgeon of his generation. He taught us how to examine patients and what questions to ask them.

Once, Prof. Sen asked me to examine a patient with acute appendicitis. I asked the man all the right questions, thoroughly inspected him and then, directly pressed his McBurney point—the site of maximum pain in appendicitis. The patient jumped up, yelping in pain. 'You are quite a ham-handed person,' Prof. Sen told me and said that one should begin examining the patient from the area where there is no pain and then gradually move to the area where there is. I've always remembered his words and followed his advice. Besides running the general surgery unit, Prof. Sen was also head of cardiac surgery. It was a treat to go into the cardiac theatre and watch him operate. We were never asked to scrub in the cardiac OT but the excitement and tension when the heart was exposed was thrilling. This was in 1953!

Frankly, while the term in surgery with Prof. Sen was enjoyable, educative and interesting, I found the medical term with Dr J.C. Patel insipid and boring. Perhaps that was because I didn't get to use my hands too much—I just had to see reports and write histories. I'd often sneak off to the outpatient department where honorary surgeons would be seeing patients. My favourite honorary was Dr A.V. Baliga. His clinics were fascinating. He would ask a student to examine a patient (there were no CT scans or sonographies in those days!) and give a diagnosis. Then, Dr Baliga would write all the other possible diagnoses on the blackboard and logically start eliminating them one by one. Finally, he'd draw a line across the blackboard and say, 'The right diagnosis is below this line.' 'Below the line' became one of our favourite phrases for correct diagnoses.

My second surgical term was with Dr Arthur D'Sa and Dr Karmarkar as assistant chief. One patient assigned to me in that term had an unusual condition called 'plunging thyroid' because of which a round swelling would pop up in his neck whenever he swallowed. In our class were three outgoing girls with whom I was friendly. One day, I told them that I could get the patient to stroke Dr Karmarkar's bald head as he was being examined. 'What nonsense!' they exclaimed. 'Impossible!' We bet on it.

I told the patient that he was going to be examined by a sweet, bald doctor who loved having his head stroked. And sure enough, when Dr Karmarkar bent down to examine him, my patient obediently patted his head. Everyone started laughing and Dr Karmarkar angrily asked the patient what he was doing. The innocent man pointed to me and said I'd asked him to.

Luckily, all Dr Karmarkar did was look at me and say, 'Udwadia, why do you do these foolish things?' He then walked away to the next patient. On another occasion, Dr Karmarkar was annoyed with me during his rounds because my operation notes were very brief. So, the next time Dr Karmarkar came for his rounds, I described an operation he'd performed for an enlarged prostate in great detail—in fact, I had copied the description of the entire procedure from our textbook. I concluded my note saying that whereas before the surgery, the patient would pass urine so slowly that he'd take minutes to finish; now, he took only a few seconds, passing urine with the force of the 'Ganges in spate'. When Dr Karmarkar read my note, he said, 'Udwadia, why do you write such rubbish?' I kept a straight face and said, 'Sir, I've seen such a thick jet come out of him.' For years thereafter, it was an incident my batchmates never let me forget.

My second medical term was under Prof. Raghvan, whose registrar and blue-eyed boy was my elder brother Farokh. I was

not interested in medicine—I was only interested in surgery—
and occasionally even sneaked away to attend surgical OPDs
during my medical postings. Once, I had a patient with a cardiac
murmur and Prof. Raghvan asked me if I knew how many
types of murmurs there were. I replied that there were two. He
seemed surprised at the depth of my knowledge and asked me
to name them. I said the first was organic but, for the life of me,
I couldn't remember the name of the second. I looked around
desperately for help and saw my brother mouthing something
from behind the professor's back. Unfortunately, I couldn't
fathom what he meant, and in the end, having nothing better
to offer, said, 'inorganic'. All the students roared with laughter
and my brother almost tore his hair out in embarrassment.

During the obstetrics term, I enjoyed doing deliveries, even
though we could only deliver babies born at night because we
worked in college all day. We had to deliver thirty newborns
during our term, and each delivery I conducted was a joy.
Between deliveries, the registrar, Dr Narvekar, a master teacher,
took clinics. I also found the gynaecology term very interesting.
The head of this department was Dr K. Masani who lived on the
third floor of Banoo Manor, the building I lived in. Dr Masani's
lectures were at 8.30 a.m. Fortunately, he offered me lifts all
the way to the college, which was the only way I could be on
time for his lectures. But since the gynaecology OT did only
a limited number of operations—the most major ones being
hysterectomies—I much preferred the general surgery OT.

Medical school, though, wasn't all work and no play. In my
third year, I contested elections for the position of debating
secretary of the college gymkhana—the student organization
that held all extracurricular activities. I was elected, and was
responsible for organizing college debates and elocutions,

inviting guest speakers to address the students and selecting teams for inter-collegiate and inter-university competitions. In my fourth year, I stood for general secretary of the college gymkhana against my good friend, the very popular Ramesh Sanzgiri. I had little hope of beating him, but two weeks before election day (when all students voted by secret ballot) a 15-foot-long poster was put up at the college entrance. It showed the Walt Disney cartoon character Goofy pulling a long cart with other Disney characters in it holding up letters that read, 'It can ONLY be Udwadia for GS'. I wondered who'd put it up—I certainly hadn't asked anyone to. It turned out to be Dinshaw Doongaji, a friend who was one year senior to me. Dinshaw had also put up smaller posters at a number of strategic sites, canvassing for me. His creative electioneering must have turned the tide, for I won. Dinshaw went on to become one of the city's leading psychiatrists and head of psychiatry at KEM.

I also began going steady with my childhood sweetheart, Khorshed, in my fourth year. She'd attend all college functions and my friends knew her well. That year, my batch decided to do a play for College Day and persuaded Dr Sudha Mody, an ophthalmic registrar at KEM who was good at theatre, to help us. Sudha suggested Molière's farce, *The Physician in Spite of Himself*, with me playing the role of a simple woodcutter who is mistaken for a doctor and ends up being a success. We started rehearsals six weeks before D-Day and they turned out to be nerve-racking. That was partly because two of our actors couldn't pronounce words the way Sudha wanted. One boy kept saying 'pauleesh' for 'police' and the other 'theeth' for 'that'. In addition, I'd keep forgetting my lines, some of which were in Latin. This happened even during our performance, but I managed to improvise, speaking gibberish instead of

Latin till the prompter woke up. The audience didn't suspect a thing and loved us.

During the final year, the only thought in our minds was the final MBBS. We had to clear both practical and theory exams in seven subjects: medicine, surgery, obstetrics and gynaecology, ophthalmology, pathology, jurisprudence and hygiene. The year was spent either in the wards, seeing and presenting cases to the registrars in the evenings, or in the pathology museum examining specimens or studying late into the night. My main goal was to ensure that I ranked in the top six of my surgical batch because my future depended on it. Without a doubt, this was the most stressful exam I had ever appeared for.

Before we knew it, five glorious, educative, fun-filled years were coming to an end. By standing fourth in surgery from my batch, I was assured of getting positions as both houseman and registrar at KEM. I looked forward to my future as a surgeon with anticipation. After the thorough training, education and hands-on experience GS Medical College and KEM Hospital had given us over five years, we simply had to make good and bring credit to our alma mater. If we did not, the onus was on us.

4

The Foundation

Although I was supposed to start working immediately as a houseman at KEM after my MBBS, I was asked to join after six months due to a bureaucratic mix-up. Not wanting to waste time, I got a job at the Bai Jerbai Wadia Hospital for Children. Built in 1928, it was the first children's hospital in India and one of the first in the world. Today, with 400 beds and more than ninety paediatricians, it has an international reputation. Paediatric surgery is an established and booming speciality in India now, but in 1957, it was unheard of and unknown. Jerbai Wadia Hospital was a trendsetter and introduced this speciality to Indian surgery.

In the first chapter of this book, I described how, on my first day at Wadia, I operated on a ten-year-old boy—or rather, how Sister Alvares, the theatre superintendent, performed the operation for me. And how, when I went down for my rounds, the boy's parents, much to my embarrassment, thanked me with tears in their eyes for saving their son's life. After my rounds, I went for lunch and found all the residents there waiting to welcome me. I was so touched. It was the beginning of a wonderful stint at Wadia. My registrar was Dr Subhash Dalal, the resident anaesthetist was Dr Shantu Vaidya and my co-house surgeon was Dr Ratan Edibam.

Subhash was an exemplary registrar. He was so meticulous during surgery and so kind to all the children that one could learn just by observing him. He taught me the importance of being gentle with all tissue during surgery, making sure that minimal tissue trauma was caused. I learnt that one could treat an adult as a big child, but not a child as a small adult. The physiology, recovery and tissue response of a child was different and demanded total gentleness and precision, a foundation I have carried all through my life from my first job, both for children and adults.

In addition to surgical duties, the housemen at Wadia also had to do basic pathology like blood counts, and urine and sugar examination. As far as possible, every member of the surgical team personally donated blood to the children as part of their duties. And if the patient had a rare blood group, there were professional donors waiting outside the hospital who were paid ₹150 each time. The house surgeons grouped and cross-matched their blood and used it only after injecting a vial of penicillin in it—a prophylaxis against sexually transmitted diseases. Today, giving blood that is not from a registered blood bank is a jailable offence, but at that time, it was quite normal.

What particularly fascinated me about Wadia's orthopedic unit was their work on 'talipes equinovarus' (club foot), a congenital abnormality in which the child is born with its foot pointing downwards and inwards. About one in a thousand children are born with a club foot, with boys being more susceptible than girls. Initial treatment consisted of stretching and manipulating the foot into the correct position and strapping and keeping it in place. It's important to start treatment as early as possible because the younger the child, the softer and more cartilaginous its bones and the easier it is to restore the normal shape of the foot.

There were so many children with this deformity that every morning, on the benches outside the theatre, there would be well over a dozen children who had come for their once-a-week strapping. This was vital; otherwise, the child would have a permanent limp, walk on the outer side of their foot, be in constant pain and remain quite miserable growing up. I took great joy in strapping these children because it was wonderful to see their deformities getting corrected.

In paediatrics, a doctor gets to see diseases not seen in adults—congenital problems such as cleft lips, cleft palates, ano-rectal deformities, as well as acquired abnormalities such as intussusception. I was sad and sorry when my six months were over and I had to say farewell to the great team of fellow residents, nurses and the children. What I didn't know at the time was that I would return a few years later as an assistant consultant paediatric surgeon but, at that time, KEM Hospital beckoned me.

* * *

After an initial three months of rotating through various surgical departments, I started my house post with Dr Karmarkar, chief of surgery, and Dr D. Karanjiawala as assistant chief on 1 October 1957 and continued with them till 31 March 1958. On my very first day at work, I reached the ward at 7.30 a.m. to be met by the very annoyed registrar, Dr G.B. Parulkar. It was an operation day and I didn't know that, on such days, the house surgeon had to be in the ward at 6 a.m. to 'prep' patients who were undergoing surgery. I had to scrub the part to be operated on with soap and water, dry it, then clean it again with ether, spirit and iodine. Finally, the cleaned part was covered with a sterile towel kept in place with bandages until the patient was moved to the operation table. To give you an idea of the extent of the prep work, there would be about seven to ten cases per operation day, spread over the male, female and children's wards. The surgeries would start at 8 a.m., and since there was a very tiny window between 'prep' and surgery, getting breakfast was always a scramble.

It was gruelling work—early to rise, late to sleep. For an allotted bed strength of thirty-five patients, we had, at any given time, about forty-five to sixty patients. And on days when we had emergencies—on both Saturdays and Sundays—we would have over seventy-five patients to look after. I was assisted by an intern, Dr Mapara, whom I affectionately called Major Map. He practically lived in the hospital, shared my room when he couldn't go home at night and was as good as a junior house surgeon in terms of help and efficiency.

There is a rare congenital condition known as ectopia vesicae where the patient's urinary bladder is maldeveloped and is exposed on the abdominal skin in such a way that urine dribbles out on the skin constantly, making life unbearable for the patient and the family. It is often combined with other congenital deformities, and these patients were usually left untreated. During my second month at this post, I admitted such a case. Dr Karmarkar saw him on his rounds the next day and said, 'Poor man, I wish we could help him.' We went to the post-graduate library the following day and, after a long search, found an operation described by Lowsley Johnson to correct this deformity. This was a difficult procedure for those times. The process involved reimplanting the ureters (tubes through which urine from the kidney passes to the bladder) into a pouch made from the colon, which would serve as a new bladder. One end of this pouch was required to be brought out from the anal sphincter so that the anal muscles could control both stools and urine, thus greatly improving the quality of life. The useless bladder wall on the abdomen would need to be excised and the abdominal wall had to be reconstructed. The procedure lasted an exhausting five hours. I was with the patient in the ward when he opened his eyes and the surprise and joy on his face when he could not smell urine or feel a wet abdomen made me feel that even a fifty-hour-long operation would have been worthwhile.

And then, lightning struck twice. During my fourth month, we saw a second case of ectopia vesicae—a sixteen-year-old boy from the same district in Uttar Pradesh (UP) as our previous patient. As I had assisted for the first case, I was requisitioned for the second too. We followed up the two cases for around eight weeks and Dr Karmarkar published a paper with me as a co-author. It was my first surgical publication.

Apart from surgery, what the post at KEM Hospital taught me was the ability to work on and on, twenty-four to forty-eight hours non-stop. At that time, there were a lot of burns patients at KEM Hospital and the houseman had to complete all the burns dressings before 4 p.m., when visiting hours began. I was rushing through the dressings and must have been rough and caused pain to a patient. As I was about to go to the next patient, I found that Dr Karmarkar was standing right behind me. Had he shouted, 'You ham-handed, stupid fellow, is this the way you dress the patient?' I would have quickly forgotten his words. Instead, he came up to me, put his hand on my shoulder, looked at me with his soft brown eyes and said, 'Udwadia, a surgeon must *himself* feel the patient's pain.' I have never heard a more profound definition of empathy.

On another occasion, while Dr Karmarkar was assisting me during a recurrent hernia operation, he asked me whether I'd noticed anything unusual. When I said I hadn't, he pointed out that in cases of recurrent hernia, there is always scar tissue, but in this case there was hardly any. Then he went on to say, 'The absence of scar tissue is the signature of a *gentle* surgeon.' This was what Dr Subhash Dalal, too, had taught me at Wadia—to treat every fibre of the patient's tissue with respect and care. Gentle surgeons are rewarded with good healing.

One of the greatest joys of those six months was to have Dr G.B. Parulkar, who was also my senior from GS, as my registrar. He was thorough and skillful but made his surgeries look easy. Most importantly, though, he gave a tremendous amount of operative work to the house surgeon. He was not lazy but exceptionally generous and took pride in seeing his housemen assist him and then independently perform procedures like hernias, appendectomies, haemorrhoids and duodenal perforations. By the time I had finished three months in the post, he felt confident that he could permit me to operate independently for all cases within my scope. His approach to teaching boosted my confidence and also taught me how I should be treating my house surgeons when I became a registrar.

Both my chiefs taught much more than just surgery. They taught me empathy, civility, care, compassion and to make sure that the patient was treated not as a 'case', but as a human being who could depend on the house surgeon for compassion and support. They did not pontificate but led by example. Six months is a short time, but those six months laid the foundation for my entire surgical career. I kept in touch with my KEM mentors throughout their lifetime. They not only had my respect, but also my affection.

* * *

It was a chance meeting after cricket practice with Dr Bhojraj, honorary anaesthetist at KEM, that led to my next post as an assistant to the renowned surgeon, Dr Baliga. Dr Bhojraj was also Dr Baliga's anaesthetist in private practice. Dr Bhojraj advised me that as I had a two-month gap between my KEM house post and my next post at Tata Hospital, I could utilize the two months working as Dr Baliga's assistant at his nursing home. I was delighted to accept the offer. One of the most important surgical influences of my life, Dr Baliga was born in 1904. He had a burning desire to become a surgeon from childhood. In 1920, when Mahatma Gandhi called upon all students to leave educational institutions run by the British, he joined the National School in Udupi, which was not accepted by the colonial government. Because its matriculation was not recognized, he could not do his MBBS. However, when he topped the Licentiate of College of Physicians and Surgeons (LCPS) examination at the National Medical College, Bombay, he attracted the attention of Dr J.V. Deshmukh, a surgeon at KEM, and was appointed as a house surgeon there. But Dr Baliga was not satisfied because he knew that, with his qualifications, he could never become eligible to appear for his Master of Surgery (MS) or Fellow of the Royal College of Surgeons (FRCS), and so could not become a full-fledged surgeon. He somehow raised the money to go to England, passed the London matriculation and got his Licentiate of Royal College of Physicians (LRCP), Member of the Royal College of Surgeons (MRCS) and FRCS qualifications. He returned to India in 1933 and was appointed as an honorary at KEM. He then went on to earn an international reputation. With his gentle ways and thorough demonstration of clinical examinations coupled with his logical approach to arriving at a diagnosis, I looked up to him as a master teacher. Even as an undergraduate in college, I would sneak off and attend his clinics even though I was not in his batch.

My first case with Dr Baliga was a frail Parsee lady in her nineties with an enormous kidney tumour. The only reason she was accepted for surgery was because the tumour was so large that she was finding it difficult to breathe. She had been referred to other surgeons but they'd declined to operate on her, probably because of her age. But Dr Baliga felt that she should be able to live in comfort even if she had only a few years left. Her son was a consultant at Tata Memorial Hospital and on the day of the surgery, a couple of surgeons from Tata came to the OT. After anaesthesia had been administered and she'd been positioned on her side for the removal of her kidney, one of the Tata surgeons offered Dr Baliga his help. 'No, thanks. I've got an excellent new surgeon to help me,' Dr Baliga replied. 'We should be all right.' He was, of course, referring to me. I felt both embarrassed and burdened.

The operation started off smoothly. The colon was reflected from the tumour; the kidney was completely mobilized and separated from surrounding structures and clamps were placed on the pedicle. But just as Dr Baliga was about to tighten the knot of the ligature on the clamp I was holding, it slipped and there was a massive gush of blood. Without saying a word, Dr Baliga put a large abdominal mop into the bleeding area and put the full pressure of his small body on it. He turned around and continued talking with the surgeons from Tata as if nothing had happened, but all the while, maintained the pressure on the bleeding area. Neither his body language nor his facial expressions suggested that he was angry with me. In fact, his sparkling eyes seemed to be smiling.

I was waiting for a dressing down, but he didn't say a word. After what seemed like an eternity, he stopped pressing down on the mop. By now, the flow of blood had considerably reduced and the bleeding vessel was visible. Dr Baliga gently put a clamp on it, gave the clamp to me and tied the ligature. Throughout, he acted as if nothing untoward had happened though, of course, the other surgeons present must have been horrified. The kidney was removed, the incision closed, the dressing applied and the patient placed on her back. Everybody relaxed when Dr Bhojraj said that the patient was doing well.

Dr Baliga took the Tata surgeons for a cup of coffee while I remained in the theatre, monitoring the patient. Finally, she was sent to her room and the next case was placed on the table.

As Dr Baliga and I were scrubbing for that operation, Dr Baliga came close to me, stood on tiptoe because he was rather short, and whispered in my ear, 'Udwadia, we must not make a habit of this.'

Those half-joking words were his only admonition. They brought home the fact that the responsibility for any surgical mishap is the surgeon's. The buck stops with them. They must always maintain their composure, ensuring the team responds with optimal efficiency. Those words also taught me that a gentle reprimand was far more effective than an angry tongue-lashing. 'Udwadia, we must not make a habit of this' has remained with me forever as the right way of dealing with my assistants if they make a mistake. If you want the loyalty of your juniors, you must give them yours first.

Another lesson he taught me was equally unforgettable. At about 11 one night, I got a call asking me to come immediately to Dr Baliga's nursing home. The patient was the wife of a KEM consultant, the leading orthopaedic surgeon of his day. It was a case of an acute abdomen. And since the orthopaedic surgeon was popular, some other KEM consultants had also come to support the couple during their ordeal.

The surgery was successfully completed in an hour, following which all of us had tea until around 2 a.m. Dr Baliga then took me aside and said that he would be flying off to Calcutta at 6 a.m. to operate on his patients there early next morning and would be back late the following evening. In the meanwhile, I was to manage the case and make sure the patient was comfortable. Since there were no surgeries during Dr Baliga's absence, I went out with Khorshed after morning rounds until 6 p.m. in the evening, and subsequently returned to his clinic to check in on all the patients, especially this lady.

She was fine, nil by mouth (she wasn't allowed to drink or eat), was passing urine freely and had a soft abdomen.

Dr Baliga called his secretary that evening to say that his return would be delayed by a day since the caseload in Calcutta was heavy. Even though I was taking care of the patient, the delay upset the KEM consultants who were coming to the clinic every evening to see their colleague's wife. I did my best to reassure them. I re-examined her, and showed them the pathology and urine reports. Everything was perfect, but they weren't satisfied. Then, to my great dismay, Dr Baliga called again to say that he was further delayed by another day. That was the last straw. The consultants were furious, insisting that I was too junior a doctor to be able to provide proper post-operative care.

Finally, on the third day, Dr Baliga arrived at about 6 p.m. I immediately requested him to first meet the consultants before he started seeing his patients. Dr Baliga's secretary must have told him that we were having a rough time in his absence, but he insisted on seeing his patients first. He had a bit of a stubborn streak. Finally, at about 8.30 p.m., I barged into his room and said, 'Sir, please show your face to all the visitors because the consultants are waiting for you. They are not going home until you meet them.'

Dr Baliga slammed his pen on the table, got up, took me by the arm and starting walking. He suddenly stopped in the corridor, three doors away from her room, made me face him and said, 'Udwadia, I am surprised at you.'

I replied, 'Sir, I did the best I could.'

'I know you did,' he said, 'but why didn't you tell them that the time for post-operative care is on the operation table, and that Dr Baliga has already done the post-operative care?'

I was stunned by the intensity of that statement.

'The time for post-operative care is on the operation table.'

I had never heard a more succinct summing up of post-operative care. As a teacher, I have repeated his words to every one of my students and feel they should be put up in every operating theatre.

Dr Baliga walked into the room with a benign smile. By that time, he'd acquired a full set of false teeth and this time, his smile was just as false as his teeth. Looking innocently at the consultants, he asked the patient if she had had dinner. She replied that she had. 'Then I will see you tomorrow morning,' he said, turned around and left.

Because I was at Dr Baliga's clinic from 7.30 a.m. to 8 p.m. every evening, I had very little time to spend with Khorshed. Sunday was Dr Baliga's busiest day—he'd operate in theatres in different city hospitals, starting at 7.30 a.m. at his nursing home. He would complete the case and rush to the next OT where a second anaesthetist and assistant would keep the case ready. After that, he would be back to the next case kept ready at the nursing home, working non-stop for at least twelve hours. I do not know if and when he had his lunch or tea, but he made sure his team was well-looked-after. It helped that the traffic on Sundays was very light in 1958.

Dr Baliga and I sometimes used to have arguments—on politics. He was one of the very few people who honestly believed in communism as a way of life. Paradoxically, he also strongly believed in freedom of speech and of the press. He believed in communism for the community and democracy for the individual. I, on the other hand, believed in complete democracy. But Dr Baliga had an open mind and would patiently listen to what I had to say. He also had a generous heart—he gave away a large part of his income towards establishing colleges, including Kasturba Medical College in Manipal.

I learnt more in two months working with Dr Baliga than I would have in one year with any other surgeon. He gave the impression of being a slow surgeon, but when you looked at the clock, the time he took was the usual for that procedure. His movements were choreographed and precise. He once told me that speed could never take precedence over precision. Some surgeons are naturally fast; but speed for the sake of it is bad surgical practice and not conducive to safe surgery. It's one of his many teachings that has always stayed with me. He lived simply and dressed modestly. Although he was a doyen of Indian surgery—looked up to by surgeons the world over—he had the kindness to mentor a young surgeon like me. He walked in the footsteps of Sushruta.

* * *

It was a tragedy that led to the construction of not only the largest cancer hospital in the country but one of the most renowned in the world. Sir Dorabji Tata's wife Meherbai died in 1932 after she had been treated for leukemia abroad. Heartbroken, her husband was determined to start a hospital that would treat cancer patients from all socio-economic classes. Towards this end, he created the Sir Dorabji Tata Trust, a substantial charitable trust that carries out tremendous philanthropic work even today. The Tata Memorial Hospital was constructed entirely through this trust and commissioned in 1941. By the time I joined in 1958, it had patients from not only every nook and corner of India but from neighbouring countries too. Its OPD load was so heavy that it was impossible to look after every patient with the care they deserved. On the other hand, its operating theatres were run with great precision.

In the 1950s, radical surgery was the primary treatment for all malignancies. Tata Memorial had just four units, four consultants, four registrars and four house surgeons. Dr Meherhomjee, Dr Jussawalla, Dr Paymaster and Dr Borges headed the four units and I was Dr Paymaster's houseman. Because there was so much work in my unit, there was hardly any opportunity for teaching. But whenever I could snatch some time, I went to see Dr Borges operate. It was a delight to watch the grace and precision with which he worked. Watching him do a radical mastectomy was almost like reading poetry. Though the procedure was ghastly from the patient's point of view, he made it look dignified and clean. During rounds, he took the time to talk to every patient, listen to them, cheer them up, and had more time for the poor than the rich.

But, for me, the atmosphere at Tata Memorial was gloomy and sad. Treatments for cancer were not as advanced then and researchers were still trying to understand what they were up against. It was sad to see patients suffering, knowing that there was no hope, and watching them die. The only chemotherapy available at that time was nitrogen mustard and I often felt that the treatment was worse than the disease.

Two patients left an indelible memory. The first was a case of cancer of the thyroid which had grown so large that it was obstructing the windpipe. Late one night, I had just finished a tracheostomy (placing an airway in an obstructed trachea or windpipe due to external pressure) when another patient, seen by Dr Jussawalla's unit previously, was rushed into the OT. He was struggling to breathe and was turning blue. His eyes were bulging and his pulse was racing. The theatre attendant tried to hold him steady as I put in a laryngoscope and sucked out the thick mucus and froth until I could see his vocal cords. I then tried using a paediatric endotracheal tube but it was met with total resistance a short distance below the vocal cords. Seconds were ticking by; the patient could die any moment. I asked the nurse for the more rigid, metal paediatric bronchoscope. She said it wasn't sterile, but I had no choice. I pushed the bronchoscope between the cords but it didn't work either. The patient suddenly stopped struggling and became lifeless. I rammed the bronchoscope in aiming for the midline, and it grated through the obstruction and opened the airway! The patient began breathing again. Oxygen was given through the scope, and his colour began improving as did his pulse. At first, I was focused on monitoring the patient and keeping the scope in position. But when I finally looked at his face, I couldn't take my eyes off him. He couldn't say anything because of the rigid scope. But he was talking with his eyes, repeating the words, 'thank you'. I was wondering how long I could keep the scope in his throat when, fortunately, Dr Jussawalla's surgical registrar came into the OT. With great relief, I handed over his case to him. I patted the patient's cheek before I left and our eyes spoke. I told him that now that his surgeon had come, all would be well. The registrar, using the bronchoscope as an airway, managed a tricky tracheostomy just above the sternum. I learnt later that the patient had extensive metastatic disease (metastasis is the spread of the cancer to several other organs). When I went to meet him, he looked very dejected. I could not help asking myself if it would have been better if he had died on my table. I thus learnt early on in my career that there can be a flip side to doing the right thing.

The other case was that of a burly butcher. He had a grossly advanced lymphoma—a lymph node malignancy in the chest cavity between the lungs in the mediastinum—which was compressing the surrounding structures. He was receiving radiation therapy with poor or no response. He was put on nitrogen mustard treatment. I never saw any of his relatives and he was always happy to talk to me on my nightly rounds. One night, I saw that the nurse had started nasal oxygen for him as he had laboured breathing and his nails were turning blue. I sat on the chair next to his bed as I did every night and he asked for a favour. Would I please give him the nitrogen mustard now rather than the next day as per schedule? He felt it would make his breathing better. I was reluctant because his veins were hard to locate in the dark ward and if the injection was not given perfectly, the consequences would be disastrous. However, he persisted and I finally agreed. Fortunately, I got a good vein. I was about to get up when he requested me to sit with him for some more time. Holding my hand tightly, he mumbled softly, with long pauses, about his work and his family in Uttar Pradesh. After a while, I tried to take away my hand, but he gripped it tighter and continued pouring out his feelings. His soft voice had a hypnotic effect. I had had a very heavy day and dozed off. I'm not sure how long I slept, but when I woke, he was quiet. I was covered in sweat, the ward was dark and silent, and my hand was still clutched tight in his. When I tried to disengage my hand from his grip, I realized that it was my hand that was gripping his now limp hand. It gave me an eerie feeling. He had stopped breathing. Every night, he would tell me that he was afraid of being alone. That night, thankfully, there was someone next to him when he died.

Tata was my fourth surgical posting after graduation. I saw, did and learnt a fair amount of oncological surgery. By the time I had finished, I had a foundation and interest in onco-surgery which has continued over the decades. Today, cancer treatment has become multidisciplinary. Surgery, from being radical and extensive, is now becoming more and more conservative—saving organs is a vital part of treatment. There are now myriad chemotherapies, each specific for a particular malignancy. There have been refinements in radiation therapy, hormone-based therapy, immune therapy, stem cell therapy and other treatment modalities, all of which combine to create a far brighter picture of the war against cancer. There is now a stronger feeling—in the profession and among patients—that the battle against cancer can be won.

5

Research

Just when there were about three weeks left for me to finish my posting at Tata, my friend Narian Chhabria, who was working in the Experimental Surgery Department at KEM, told me that Prof. Sen wanted to meet me right away. So, the next day, I walked across from Tata to KEM. Prof. Sen said that the Indian Council of Medical Research (ICMR) had approved his research projects and had asked him to select a young surgeon who could work on them for a fellowship. He had selected me. The fellowship required me to work in collaboration with Dr Chhabria on two projects, as well as one on myocardial revascularization—which is improving the circulation of blood in the heart—that I had to do on my own.

My project was titled BIMAL or Bilateral Internal Mammary Artery Ligation. Prof. Sen postulated that since the internal mammary artery has a large branch (pericardiophrenic branch) where the pericardial vessels anastomosed with the myocardial vessels, if the artery was ligated below the branch, all the blood would be diverted to the pericardiophrenic vessels thus increasing flow to the anastomosis and, perhaps, increasing myocardial flow too. In simple terms, if we closed the internal mammary artery, the blood would have nowhere to go and would be diverted into the terminal branches of the pericardial vessels which anastomose with the terminal branches of the cardiac vessels, thereby improving cardiac circulation. This procedure was akin to building a dam to divert the flow of the river.

The fellowship was godsent. I was planning to get married in a few weeks and it would be wonderful to have an eight-to-five job with no emergency duties. Moreover, it would give me ample opportunity to study for my MS which I was planning to take in May 1960. And since I'd be at KEM, I could occasionally take some time off research to attend clinics, go to OTs to see surgeries being done there and generally keep my hand in. Best of all, I'd earn twice as much than I would have as a house surgeon. And, to a newly married couple, every extra rupee was welcome!

Today, every cardiologist and cardiac surgeon is familiar with coronary artery bypass grafting surgery as well as stenting, but to think of myocardial revascularization in 1958 shows how far-thinking Prof. Sen was. He was obsessed with improving myocardial circulation in patients with coronary artery disease and I was pleased and proud to be a part of what he was trying to achieve.

My job entailed going to the morgue every day and, using a fresh, unclaimed body, dissecting the internal mammary artery. This was not easy. For starters, the procedure had to be done on a low table in a tiny area next to the noisy post-mortem room. Secondly, the lighting was very poor. Finally, the dissection itself would be tricky, given the narrow space between the second and third ribs, and the artery being deep inside, behind the chest muscles. Once the artery was identified, it had to be tied off on both left and right sides between the second and third intercostal space in the belief that, due to the anastomosis between the end branches of the pericardial and cardiac vessels, the flow to the myocardium would be increased.

BIMAL was based on an anatomical fact but it was still theoretical. The anastomosis between the two end vessels had to be captured on an X-ray plate by a portable X-ray machine after injecting dye into it. Capturing the minute vessels would require pinpoint setting of the machine. Mr Khan, the assistant for this ICMR project, and I had to do this by trial and error. In those days, the hazards of radiation were not taken seriously. And since we didn't have an X-ray technician, it took us quite a while to figure out the exact settings. This was required to be done on several cadavers. Neither Khan nor I were provided with lead shields and were exposed to considerable radiation. That could perhaps be the reason why I developed cancer of the thyroid many years later.

After I'd worked for three months on cadavers, Prof. Sen decided that it was time we tried BIMAL on patients who had undergone myocardial infarction (significantly reduced blood flow to the heart) and were deteriorating in spite of being under medical treatment—but only after we'd obtained their informed consent. Their internal mammary artery was ligated between the second and third intercostal junction on both sides under local anaesthesia. A cardiologist then followed up with them over the next few months. At the end of the year, we did a statistical study on our results for both cadavers and humans. Though Prof. Sen felt that there was some merit in the procedure, it was quite inconclusive and frankly, to me, unsubstantiated. Our study was published and presented at the annual meeting of the Cardiac Society as Bombay with Dr Rustom Jal Vakil, the famous cardiologist, as the chair.[*] After I had made the presentation, Dr Vakil asked me my opinion of the results. I replied that the results were inconclusive but that the study had been worth doing. Dr Sen didn't say anything. Dr Vakil said that if he were to snip off a small piece from the patient's earlobe, the results would be the same. I was very hurt by his sarcasm. I told him that even if a study does not give fruitful results, if it was done honestly, it was worthwhile. Dr Vakil apologized and said that while he appreciated our methodology, he doubted if it could ever improve myocardial circulation. Subsequent work by other researchers proved that Dr Vakil was right.

I then teamed up with Dr Chhabria on the next two research projects. Both were concerned with finding a safe way to do open-heart surgery. The first one involved finding the optimal concentration of potassium chloride solution that could be injected into the coronary arteries to cause cardiac arrest but, at the same time, allowed surgery on the still heart and then got the heart to resume normal functioning. Too much

---

[*] P.K. Sen, T.E. Udwadia, T.P. Kulkarni and S.G. Kinare, 'Bilateral Internal Mammary Artery Ligation for Coronary Heart Disease,' *Indian Heart Journal*, 1960.

potassium chloride could kill a patient, and too little would be ineffective. To do this, we worked with dogs. We had to open a dog's chest, dissect the aorta at its root, cross-clamp it and inject the potassium solution so that it flowed into the coronary arteries and caused cardiac arrest. The dog's heart then had to be opened and closed as for an open-heart procedure. The post-arrest recovery of the heart was carefully monitored in terms of rhythm abnormalities, strength of myocardial function and other parameters, after which the chest was closed.

Our second joint project was to determine if deep hypothermia—or cooling of the entire body which, incidentally, cools the heart—could be used to induce cardiac arrest long enough for reconstructive heart surgery and normal cardiac recovery. We had to anaesthetize a dog, intubate it and keep it on a pump ventilator. We then had to apply ECG leads and immerse the dog in a tub of ice, salt and water. Continuous rectal temperature monitoring was done. Cardiac arrest took place at around 27 degrees Celsius. The parameters we studied were: the duration of arrest, the flaccidity of the heart and the smoothness of recovery in terms of fibrillation, rhythm abnormality, ECG changes, strength of cardiac muscle contractions and so on.[*] It was a matter of joy and satisfaction to Narian and me that both our experimental studies were put to clinical use for open-heart surgery.

I must confess that, as an inveterate dog lover, it was difficult to mentally condition myself to conduct experiments on dogs. I fed them dog biscuits but that did very little to assuage my conscience. But if you have the temperament and thrust for

---

[*] P.K. Sen, N.D. Chhabria and T.E. Udwadia, 'Induced Cardiac Arrest Under Hypothermia,' *Indian Journal of Surgery*, 1960.

research, it becomes almost an addiction. The one year that I spent in KEM's research department opened my mind to a world that had nothing to do with day-to-day surgery or patient care. To come up with better ways of performing surgical procedures, better ways of solving long-standing clinical problems—what could be more exhilarating? My friends jokingly referred to me as a 'dog surgeon' but I feel that I had the last laugh. Less than 2 per cent of surgical residents in India have long-term exposure to research. I was blessed by an ICMR post being created when I was looking for a job and the fact that Prof. Sen asked me to take it. Thanks to that ICMR fellowship, I continued to carry out research throughout my career as well as expose my residents to this vital aspect of surgical training.

6

My Surgical Registrarship

Having worked for one thrilling and educative year with Prof. Sen in the research department, I was amazed at his wide and distant vision. His thinking was way beyond contemporary surgery, and contemporary surgeons. He was not just an excellent surgeon but also a surgical pioneer and philosopher. Having already worked with him in the experimental surgery lab, I realized the advantage and value of working with him for an additional two years as his registrar.

Working with him as registrar—like many fortunate occurrences in my career—was also purely by accident. Dr Sen's registrarship was the preserve of the class topper in surgery—in this case, Dr Bhadreshwar—while I stood fourth, which meant that I was slated to work with Dr Arthur D'Sa.

Just before I was to start my post, I took on a six-month stint at the Department of Anatomy, Seth GS Medical College, as an anatomy demonstrator since anatomy is the foundation of surgery. Two months into the job, I learnt that Dr Bhadreshwar had contracted tuberculosis and the second and third-ranked candidates refused to accept Prof. Sen's registrarship as it was considered a very heavy responsibility. To my great joy, by this series of accidents, I was offered a job with Prof. Sen starting 1 March 1960. The professor of anatomy, Prof. Bhatnagar, gracefully permitted me to resign as anatomy demonstrator so that I could take up the post.

All my friends advised me to turn down the offer as the two previous applicants had done. Their argument was that the job involved not one but two surgical departments—general surgery and thoracic surgery—which was double the workload. I was planning to do my MS in May and my wife was expecting our first child; all of which could lead to personal and professional conflicts. But I knew that this was an opportunity of a lifetime and since Khorshed was due in February and staying with her mother for a few months after the delivery, I could start my post in March, giving me time to settle down in the resident quarters. An added attraction was that Dr G.B. Parulkar, the registrar during my house post with Dr Karmarkar, was now the lecturer in Prof. Sen's unit.

Prof. Sen had two units under him in Ward V of KEM Hospital—the general surgery unit and the cardiovascular/ thoracic surgery unit. There was one houseman, Dr Sharad Pandey and one registrar—me—to look after both units. The unit had a set routine: two days were devoted to the general surgery OT, two days to the cardiovascular surgery OT, one day for the OPD and emergency services where the registrar and housemen would operate all night on emergency cases and Saturday was reserved for experimental surgery where we worked with dogs. This meant that the registrar would operate six days a week, a dream come true for any surgeon who wanted to build a strong foundation. After the thoracic list ended at 1 p.m. on Friday, the 'grand round' in Ward V would start at 2 p.m., which Prof. Sen's postgraduates, the cardiology chief and residents would attend, making it a large crowd. This was a detailed round during which every patient was discussed, and would go on past 4.30 p.m. Prof. Sen had a few personal and professional idiosyncrasies. Personally, he was very friendly and understanding of his research fellows but rather suspicious of his clinical registrars and housemen. I realized this because I had worked both as his research fellow and his registrar. Professionally, he was convinced that all duodenal perforations close spontaneously and did not require surgery. This was completely contrary to clinical evidence. He had given strict instructions to his residents that duodenal perforations—one of the commonest emergencies—were not to be operated upon.

Prof. Sen's ward was Ward V and each ward had two units separated by a wide passage in the middle. The other unit in Ward V was that of Dr Vasant Sheth which was essentially a Gastro-Intestinal (GI) surgery unit. Prof. Sen's unit consisted of him as head of the department of surgery and head of cardiovascular surgery, Dr T.P. Kulkarni as assistant professor, Dr G.B. Parulkar as lecturer, myself as registrar and Sharad Pandey as house surgeon. GB, I knew already because he was my registrar when I was house surgeon to Dr Karmarkar and we got on like a house on fire. I was the common registrar for both general surgery and thoracic surgery and was hence expected to know everything about every patient during rounds. During routine rounds, Prof. Sen would ask questions and discuss cases with the house surgeon and undergraduate students. However, on grand rounds, all questions and discussions were directed towards the registrar.

On a grand round, three months into my post, a patient from Dr Vasant Sheth's side of the ward (where we were trying to hide him) came over; lifted up his hospital coat, stood in front of me and said, *'Sahab, taaka kabhi nikalega? Char baje humko janeka hai* (Sir, when will you remove my stitches? I have to leave at 4).' I told him to wait, saying that they would be removed in time. Dr Sen raised his eyebrows but carried on. The patient came back a little later and this time, he forcefully demanded that I remove the stitches. That's when Prof. Sen asked, 'Udwadia, why is Vasant Sheth's patient telling you what to do?'

I had no option but to tell him the truth. I said that his was a case of duodenal perforation. The patient came three days after perforation and was operated upon seven days ago. Duodenal perforation was one of the commonest emergencies in the 1950s, 1960s and 1970s. A duodenal perforation is an ulcer which gradually penetrates the wall of the duodenum (the part of the intestine where the stomach with its acid juice and food empties into). The contents of the stomach and bile leak through the hole into the peritoneal cavity, causing an inflammation of the cavity. He flared up, 'You have an order not to operate on duodenal perforations. Why did you do it?' I explained that this was a high-risk case that had come to us three days after the perforation and I felt that the patient could die if he was not operated upon urgently. He didn't buy this argument and accused me of operating just for the sake of it. I replied that the surgery hadn't been carried out by me but by the houseman, Dr Pandey. He asked why I had let the houseman operate. In the presence of over twenty doctors on the round, I too lost my temper and replied that I had pride in my houseman. It was my duty to train him properly, and if he couldn't operate on a simple duodenal perforation, one of the most common surgical emergencies, he would be a laughing stock. The registrar's position at KEM is a teaching position. I also told him that I had a duty towards my patient. Dr Sen left the round in a huff and sent for me to come to his office.

I knew that this was the tipping point of my registrarship. If I rubbed him the wrong way, I could be asked to leave, but if I kept quiet, he would bully me for the remainder of my post. When I went to his office, he said, 'Udwadia, I have worked with you and I did not expect this from you.' I told him it was my duty as a doctor to have this perforation sutured, otherwise the patient could have died. I also added that those who were not in danger were conserved, as he must have seen on his rounds but emergencies were emergencies.

After a long pause, he asked 'Udwadia, who is the chief of this unit, you or me?' After a pause, I said that it was a difficult question to answer, which made him smile. I finally said, 'Of course, you, sir. But I have an obligation towards my patient and my house surgeon.' I could see him relax. He relented, saying I could be permitted to operate on extreme cases, but that he needed to know beforehand. I replied that it would not be pleasant for him because I would be phoning him up every emergency night.

Our skirmish ended in a draw. Neither side won, but we both knew that he could not push me around. I thought that this confrontation might harm my career, but on the contrary,

Prof. Sen's attitude towards me changed completely. He was more affable and ready to listen to me. From that moment on, we hit it off.

Sharad Pandey, my house surgeon for the first six months, was the best houseman I had ever worked with. He was very easy-going and cheerful but also disciplined and could work twenty-four hours without complaint. One patient, a municipal sewer cleaner, taught us never to take a duodenal perforation lightly. He came on our Thursday emergency day with a duodenal perforation, frank peritonitis. Sharad operated on him while I assisted and the procedure went well. Exactly a week later, on Thursday, he reperforated and I sutured him this time. The patient had a big, twisted moustache and Sharad warned him that he would shave it off if he perforated again. The following Thursday, like clockwork, he reperforated and GB sutured him. And . . . you guessed it, he reperforated exactly one week later. He'd been in the ward for three weeks, had been operated upon thrice and was going downhill.

I realized that merely re-suturing the perforation would be a waste of time and that he needed a more radical procedure. I discussed this with other registrars in the quarters and the unanimous opinion was that he needed a sub-total gastrostomy which entailed the removal of two-thirds of his distal (the lower part) stomach, a duodenal closure and a gastrojejunostomy, which involved joining the remaining stomach to the small intestine so that food from the stomach could move forward. A registrar, Dr Patel, who later became head of urology at Sion Hospital, volunteered to assist Sharad and me. Dr S. Shah, whom I was comfortable with, was the anaesthetist. With two units of blood, we took him up for surgery which lasted about three hours. We kept him in the OT till the morning as that was next best to a non-existent Intensive Care Unit (ICU). The patient went home twelve days after surgery. His prized twisted moustache was untouched. It is believed that bankers, lawyers and the wealthy have high acidity levels and ulcers because they are stressed. There can be no greater cause of stress than not knowing where your next meal will come from!

One day a month, the entire surgical department, including the chiefs of all six units, all assistant chiefs, residents as well as undergraduate and postgraduate students, came together for the 'death conference' where all units would report on every death in their unit for that month to a packed lecture hall. Deaths were divided into four categories: the first was patients' disease (PD) where the patient already came in with a condition that could not be salvaged. The second was error in diagnosis (ED) where the unit had misdiagnosed the case, leading to the patient's death. The third was error of management (EM) where the diagnosis had been right, but the treatment or surgery had not resulted in the patient getting saved. The fourth category was God Only Knows or GOK. After fierce argument and discussion, each unit would try to categorize the death into either PD or GOK and the respective chiefs would defend their residents saying that the cause of death was not preventable. This conference was a matter of great rivalry between the six units.

The only unit where the chief would criticize his own residents was ours. Prof. Sen would try his best to show that the death was due to an error of diagnosis or error of management, which obviated the need for the other chiefs to argue because he would do that on their behalf. We would wind up fighting among ourselves. After every death conference, Sharad and I would be pretty mad at Prof. Sen for not backing us up unlike the other unit heads. Eventually, we hit upon a plan to strike back.

Once every few months, Prof. Sen would invite the whole unit and their spouses to his house for dinner. It was an enjoyable affair because his wife Marie was a warm, friendly hostess. Sen had a very strange house spread over four levels. The living room was on the ground floor, the dining room on the first, his study was on the second floor and his bedroom on the third. The telephone was downstairs, between the dining and living rooms. After a particularly brutal death conference, Sharad and I—after finishing our ward work at around 1 or 2 in the morning—would telephone him, make him come all the way downstairs to answer the phone and hang up after hearing him say, 'Hello, Hello, Hello' repeatedly! This would give us immense joy.

There was one horror-filled night when we lost three cardiac patients between 11 p.m. and 3 a.m. While they were operated upon on different days, they all died on the same night and we were up all night trying to resuscitate them, sympathizing with their relatives, filling death certificates and finding an appropriate cause of death. In the early 1960s, there was no ICU. However major the procedure or poor the state of the patient or severe the post-operative complications, they were all kept in the general ward. If they needed ventilation, we had to ventilate them using an Ambu bag, which is a rubber bag the size of half a football that had to be squeezed sixteen times a minute to help the patient breathe. I don't think anyone, be it our chiefs, the relatives or the nurses, ever understood the trauma, stress and guilt the residents carried when patients didn't make it, even though we were not responsible for their deaths. Just as I resolved never to be an onco-surgeon after seeing the agony of patients at Tata Memorial Hospital, I told Sharad as we walked back to the RMO quarters at 6 a.m. that I would never become a cardiac surgeon. But circumstances bring out different reactions in different people. His response was the opposite—because of that night, he said he *would* become a cardiac surgeon. And he did.

After passing my Fellowship of the College of Physicians and Surgeons (FCPS) exam in April, a month after I joined Prof. Sen's team, I was planning to take the MS exam in May. Sen tried to persuade me to postpone taking the exam in May, telling me that my son was born in February; I started the registrarship in March, I did the FCPS in April and wanted to do the MS in May. He felt that I was trying to grab too much all at one time. I explained to him that if I did my MS in May, I would be able to concentrate only on surgery for the rest of my registrarship. He said, 'You do what you like, but I must remind you that in May, the MS examination will be at JJ Hospital.' There was a sinister significance to his words, because those were the years of the interminable 'Great War' between KEM and JJ.

Khorshed and Rushad (my son) were still at her mother's house so there was no one at home. The theory exams went off without a hitch and on the day of the MS practical exam, which was to be held at JJ, I was at home in the morning, hoping that I would get phone calls wishing me luck. Khorshed, of course, called, but I was hoping I would get a call from my brother Farokh. I used to drive him to all his exams, be they the MBBS, FCPS or MD. But he didn't call, which depressed me. My first practical exam consisted of short cases which were very straightforward. The first case was of a fourteen-year-old boy with tubercule lymph nodes of the neck which were so advanced that they were a classical representation of what was shown in Das's book on clinical surgery. But I could not examine him the way I'd have liked to because there was no empty bed for him to lie on for me to examine his abdomen. He was seated on a stool, waiting for his examination. I diagnosed him, nonetheless.

When I was examining my third case, I could see my examiner, a well-built Sikh gentleman with a grey beard and a red turban, walking towards me. He asked me what my diagnosis was, pointing to the first patient, the boy with the tubercule lymph nodes. I replied that it was a case of tuberculous cervical lymphadenitis. He asked if I had examined the spleen. I replied that I was waiting to finish my examination of the third case and then I'd put this boy on the bed to examine the spleen. He then remarked that if I had not examined the spleen, how could I make a diagnosis? I said that I did so on inspection and palpation and that this was as classic a case of cervical tuberculosis as one could ever get. He raised his bushy eyebrows, took out a pen and wrote an F (F in the MS meant FAIL) against my name and showed me the remark.

His co-examiner told him that I still had two more cases to go before I could be given the mark. But my examiner didn't think that would make a difference because anyone who did not examine the spleen in a lymphadenopathy had no right to pass the MS. As he was walking away, he turned around and said that I could always tell my friends that I was failed by a Hunterian professor, which was a high honour given by the Royal College of Surgeons of England. He didn't examine me on the other two cases. Straight from there, I had to go for my long cases where I got a G, which is the opposite of an F, but it made no difference.

I went to the RMO quarters, locked the door and wept myself to sleep. I felt that I had let down my wife, my son and my chief. I dreamt that I pulled out the hair from the examiner's beard, strand by strand, until his face was completely hairless. I swore that although I didn't know who or what a Hunterian professor was, I would become a Hunterian professor myself. While I had a miserable night, the morning brought with it insight and clarity. I was completely at peace with myself. I realized that when I took clinics for undergraduate students on lymph nodes, I would insist that lymph nodes from all parts of the body should be palpated as also the spleen. If I had been teaching this, then I had no business not doing it myself in the MS exam. When one realizes that the cause of failure is one's own fault and one accepts the truth, failure loses its sting.

Despite asking me not to appear for the exam, Prof. Sen was surprised that I had failed. He consoled me that it was not a big deal and I would surely clear it in October. I passed the MS in October, as Prof. Sen had predicted. Two days after I passed my MS, he encouraged me to become a member of the Association of Surgeons of India (ASI); he felt that every young surgeon must do so and present papers at the annual conference. I became a member and presented a paper on intussusception at the Poona conference (1960) and on duodenal perforation at Baroda (1961). During my tenure as registrar, I was fortunate to present two papers over two consecutive years at the Association of Surgeons of India (ASI) conference, thanks to the push by Prof. Sen.

I started the second year of my registrarship in March 1961, and I found Dr Sen to be even more receptive and encouraging. I saw a different side to him as well. There was a beautiful seven-year-old girl from Kashmir who had a patent ductus arteriosus. This condition presents as a congenital abnormal connection between the aorta and the pulmonary artery so that blood is pushed away from the aorta and into the pulmonary artery, giving rise to a large number of complications, making long-term life impossible. While the parents came to Bombay because of Prof. Sen's reputation, the long and short of it is that the child died on the table. We were so traumatized with the outcome that we cancelled the rest of the list. Hours later, I knocked on Prof. Sen's door and went in. His head was down, resting on his folded arms on the table. When I entered, he looked up—his eyes were wet with tears. Behind the facade of a tough guy, he was a softie.

Prof. Sen was something of a Renaissance man. He wrote poetry, played the sitar, was an astronomer and golfer. He was also a prolific painter and dozens of his paintings were stacked all over his house. Prof. Sen was close friends with the artist K.K. Hebbar and offered me one of his works. Stupidly, I turned down the offer. Had I taken it up, the painting would have fetched a fortune. However, I did take the *Lady in the Red Dress* by Prof. Sen; it has pride of place in my home.

There was also no subject where one could get the better of him. I don't know when he got the time to read so extensively about art, literature and music. However, there was this one time when I thought I could have been one up on him. Famously reluctant to grant leave, I asked him for some time off one afternoon for my pilot's written exam. When I told him I was flying a Piper Cub, he asked, 'What will happen to your flight if the pitch of the screw of the propeller was changed by 1/28th of an inch?' I did not know if this was a trick question, but it was then that I learnt that I couldn't ever have an advantage over him. He was also a pilot.

Every year, KEM awards a prize for the best clinical research analysis for that year and I wrote on our experience of duodenal perforations.* This paper won the award, thanks largely to the statistical study done by the unit intern, Dr R. Minina. More importantly, this study was published and, to my absolute joy, it was abstracted in the *Year Book of Surgery, 1964* edited by Michael de Bakey. Outstanding surgical papers published during that year from all over the world were abstracted in the book. When I returned after my FRCS, Sen presented me with the book along with an inscription, 'Tehemton, I have gone through this book. Yours is the only paper written by a registrar!'

During the last six months of my registrarship with Prof. Sen, the surgeries I performed were comparable to any major surgery anywhere and GB would readily give me a hand. Sister Samson, the OT superintendent at KEM, ruled with an iron hand. I felt she had a soft corner for me but if she caught me at any mischief, she would grab me by my apron collar, bring her face close and with her scary, popping eyes and big nose, warn me through her broken front teeth to 'Watch it, son'.

One day, I asked Prof. Sen if he would do a general surgery case. His reply was that I never offered him a case; if I did, he would do one. I searched for the most difficult case in the ward and finally found an enormous thyroid in a female patient that I thought he may have liked to do. He requested that I assist him. I assisted him and, I must say, he did it better than many competent and well-known general

---

* T.E. Udwadia, P.K. Sen, G.B. Parulkar and A.E. Mody, 'Acute Duodenal Perforation—a Study of 317 Cases,' *Journal of Indian Medical Science*, 1962.

surgeons would have. On his good days, Prof. Prafulla Kumar Sen was a magician; on his normal days, he was excellent and very rarely did he have an off day. Looking back, I think he was very emotionally motivated.

To my great sadness, the two years were coming to an end. Having not taken a single day off, I had accumulated twenty-one days of leave which I decided to take at the end so that I could leave India to go abroad in February. I asked Prof. Sen if I could have his testimonial. He told me to tell whoever asked that I had worked as Prof. Sen's registrar for two years and both he and I had survived. He had a hearty laugh after he said that, but he gave me a flattering testimonial. The department of cardiothoracic surgery at KEM started by him is named after him. Prafulla Kumar Sen was more than a master surgeon. He was a visionary, a philosopher and the most versatile person I have ever known—an inspiration to all who worked with him, and a legend who created a generation of surgeons as his legacy. Working with him gave me the strength, vision, passion, ethical code, quiet confidence and surgical grounding for the rest of my career.

7

Veni, Vidi, Vici, Dublin, Edinburgh, Liverpool

When I was planning to take up the FRCS exam, I did some research. I found that the passing percentage for the primary FRCS was 10 per cent in London, 12 per cent in Edinburgh and about 15 per cent in Dublin. Believing in the safety of numbers, I chose to do my primary FRCS exam in Dublin, post which I could do my final exams in any of the royal colleges across the UK.

In February 1962, Khorshed and I settled down in a boarding house within an easy twenty-minute walk to the college, leaving behind my son Rushad aged two and the new addition to the family—my daughter Dinaz, aged 9 months—in the care of my in-laws. Our landlady, Mrs Kay Mills, was typically Irish, warm and friendly. Her charges for bed, breakfast and dinner were four guineas a week for each of us. Ireland is cold in February and the only way we could keep warm in our room was to keep putting money—a shilling at a time—into the gas meter.

One of the first things I noticed was the preponderance of women as compared to men, mainly due to the paucity of employment opportunities. The men had migrated, leaving the women behind. But from what I could see, they didn't seem to mind. On my way to college, I used to pass a group of women sitting on the steps in their house coats chatting away and, when I would come back late in the evening, I would see the same group talking to each other. To me, the Ireland of the early 1960s seemed laid-back and happy and the people were as warm as Indians.

The teaching at the college was quite good, particularly in anatomy. In addition to lectures, the subject was taught on a cadaver by a grumpy old man named Garry, who was a very good anatomist and had obviously been teaching for at least fifty years. He spoke very fast and it was difficult to follow him because of his accent. The physiology and biochemistry lectures were also of a good standard. The Irish Royal College was so simple and small, and its canteen so pleasant, that we soon felt at home.

The primary FRCS exam was in the first week of June. I thought I did well. The results were announced in a most unusual way. At 7 p.m., the hall porter, in his impressive uniform, came to the front door, while all the candidates stood on the pavement below, and read out the numbers of the candidates who had passed. To my great relief, my number was among them. Khorshed and I celebrated by having our first non-boarding house dinner at a small restaurant.

I'd decided to take my final FRCS in Edinburgh since it was better known and recognized in India. We sent for our children and as soon as Khorshed's parents brought them to Dublin, we left for Edinburgh. We'd made a reservation at an Edinburgh hotel, but couldn't afford to stay there for very long. We immediately started hunting for an inexpensive flat while Soli Adrianwala—my classmate from KEM who was in the city preparing for his FRCS—very kindly babysat Rushad and Dinaz. It took us three days to find an apartment that we could afford. It was filthy, had a sitting room, a dining room, a small kitchen and a bedroom with two beds. But luckily, it also had a washroom, a tub, a basin and a toilet which was very unusual, since our neighbours had to use a large block of common washrooms. Edinburgh was really quite primitive in 1962. Later, to our embarrassment, we learnt the apartment had been used as a brothel before we took it.

The rent was four guineas a week. Within a couple of days, we were able to make the apartment liveable and I started attending the Royal College. The college had a beautiful library that was nice and warm. I would take my books there and study till late evening. There were several Indians in the library and I became friendly with Dr N. Rangabashyam from Chennai. We would discuss surgery during study breaks. Tea cost six pence per cup but at an establishment about a mile away called Larry's, it was five pence. So, Ranga and I would often walk there for a cuppa to save exactly one pence.

We joined the clinical classes of Mr Gunn, a senior registrar. He was excellent and I got a good idea of how the FRCS exam in Edinburgh was held and what was expected of the candidates. Having done my MS, I was far more confident of the final FRCS than I'd been of the preliminary in Dublin.

By the first week of August, our bank balance was so low that we couldn't afford the flat we'd rented and it became clear that all four of us couldn't continue living together. So, I wrote to my in-laws, requesting them to send tickets for Khorshed and the children to return to Bombay. I would somehow manage on my own, I said. I also wrote to my friend Raja Dhurandar, my KEM roommate, about our plans. In the last week of August, I got a telegram telling me that I'd been appointed as a registrar at the Royal Liverpool Children's Hospital and had to join immediately. Of course, I thought this was a sick joke—probably played by friends who knew about my financial situation. As I hadn't applied for any job, I decided not to respond.

You can imagine my surprise when I was summoned the next day by the secretary of the Royal College of Surgeons, Mr Patterson Ross, who asked why I hadn't responded to the notification. I explained my reasons. He said that, even so, I should contact them. On calling the hospital, I was told that the post had indeed been reserved for me and that I should join immediately. I couldn't understand how I had been given a job I had not applied for. But, at any rate, I left for Liverpool and my family followed me in due course. Now that I was earning a salary, my financial crisis may have been over, but the mystery remained.

The previous registrar at the Liverpool hospital had been boarding with a Mrs Robinson and she agreed to rent the two-bedroom apartment to me. I phoned Khorshed, asking her to come with the children to Liverpool. We needed only one bedroom for the four of us, so we used the other bedroom to store our luggage. The kitchen was very small but well laid out and had all the necessary equipment. Owing to the fact that I was on call five days a week and had to get to the hospital at short notice any time of the day or night, I also bought the cheapest second-hand car I could find for the princely sum of £110.

Heating in the apartment was by an open coal fire. It took Khorshed a long time to learn how to light a fire and get it going. There were times when I thought that she would set the whole house ablaze. Once the fire in the bedroom was lit and stable, it was wonderfully warm.

Work at the Liverpool Children's Hospital was very interesting and very productive. I had two chiefs—Mr Peter Rickham and Miss Forshall. Mr Rickham, who had given me the job, was a brilliant surgeon, a fabulous thinker and very progressive, but also very demanding. His special area of interest was hydrocephalus (where a large amount of cerebrospinal fluid in the brain compresses the brain tissue, causing deterioration of function and a very swollen head). Mr Rickham would surgically reduce the fluid in the brain thereby preserving the brain tissue to help the child lead a normal life. He would put a Pudenz valve outside the brain that drained the cerebrospinal fluid into the jugular vein in the neck. I enjoyed the operation and very soon, Mr Rickham permitted me to do it independently.

The other consultant, Miss Forshall, was an elderly lady, very prim and proper. On the days of her rounds, she would arrive promptly at 8 a.m. in her Bentley. She'd do the same surgery she'd been doing for several decades. She used to do one thing that annoyed me no end. Every time we started a round, she would greet me but deliberately mispronounce my name. She would turn to me and say, 'Good morning, Mr Udwadarrr.' I would correct her saying, 'It's Udwadia, Miss Forshall.' The next day, it would be Mr Udchkara, and so on. After tolerating this for about two months, the straw that broke the camel's

71

back was the day she called me, 'Mr Udwajichka', whatever that meant. I replied, 'It's Mr Udwadia, Miss Foreskin!' There was dead silence in the room but the message was loud and clear. Although I felt quite bad about the incident later on, I was Mr Udwadia from that day onward. Clearly, some English people still felt that India was their colony.

The mystery of my job offer was about to be solved. Three months into my Liverpool post, an American paediatric surgeon named Dr Koop—who eventually become the surgeon general of the United States and was responsible for the campaign against tobacco—visited Mr Rickham. The three of us were having lunch when Dr Koop asked me, 'How's your chief?' Puzzled, I looked at Mr Rickham.

'No, no,' Dr Koop said. 'I don't mean Peter. I mean your chief in Bombay, P.K. Sen.'

'He's well,' I replied, 'but why do you ask?'

Dr Koop said Prof. Sen and he were good friends and that, some months earlier, PK had phoned Koop and told him that one of his boys was in financial trouble in England and requested Koop to find a good registrar's job for him in England as soon as possible. That's when I understood how I'd got a registrar's job at the Royal Liverpool without having applied for it. It was then that I realized that a chief must look after his residents forever.

The Edinburgh FRCS theory exam was on 3 January 1963. That year had been the worst winter in the UK in sixty years. There was no direct train connection between Liverpool and Edinburgh and I had to change trains midway. As I left Liverpool on 2 January, a snow plough train was clearing the tracks ahead of mine. On reaching Edinburgh, I checked into a hotel as close to the college as possible for the night. The next morning, I completed both papers and caught a train back to Liverpool in the evening.

I had to change trains at a station called Carstairs. The platform had no roof and it was snowing. On seeing a telephone booth on the platform, I immediately dashed inside to keep warm. As I stood shivering inside, another passenger who'd also got off at Carstairs came and stood outside the booth. I felt sorry and invited him in. Twenty minutes later, the London train arrived and both of us scrambled into a wonderfully warm and clean second-class carriage.

A week later, the practical exam was conducted in Edinburgh in a very friendly and warm atmosphere. And then, at 7 p.m., along with the other candidates, I stood on the pavement as the hall porter read out the results. I'd passed! I immediately phoned Khorshed with the good news.

The next morning was my operation day. I could not take more than a day's leave, otherwise I'd have lost a day's salary. As soon as I entered the OT, I was asked what had happened. I gave a thumbs up and the entire staff cheered.

Till then, I had been called Dr Udwadia, but the moment I passed the FRCS, I became Mr Udwadia, the honorific for all surgeons in the UK. This strange British practice arose because in the eighteenth century, physicians were required to study at a university whereas surgeons were not. Surgeons were considered tradesmen who learnt their trade by being apprenticed to a more senior practitioner. Physicians who'd completed their university training were entitled to be addressed as 'doctor', whereas surgeons had to be content with 'mister'. Of course, with time, these arrangements changed and surgeons had to go to university too. But the British are great lovers of tradition, so surgeons continue to be referred to as 'mister'.

Open fires were the only way of keeping a house warm in Liverpool at that time, and burns were among the most common cases involving children that we had to handle in the hospital. Once, after I had finished an extensive burn grafting on a seven-year-old girl, the anaesthetist seemed very perturbed. I asked her what the problem was. She said that while she was removing the plastic tube which had been passed through a needle to start the intravenous, a part of it had been left behind in the child's vein. I had X-rays taken with dye and we found that the plastic was in the left subclavian vein, and about to enter the innominate vein. From there, it could easily slip into the child's heart, becoming a major medico-legal issue.

The anaesthetist immediately called her husband, a prominent lawyer. He advised her that a senior surgeon should handle the case. The girl was Mr Rickham's patient and I immediately called him. But since he was handling a major case at another children's hospital, there was no way he could come, and I had to do my best. Remembering my work with Prof. Sen, I opened the subclavian between two black silk loops and under screening control, put in a forceps, caught the plastic tube inside the chest, withdrew it and closed the opening in the subclavian vein. To our relief, all turned out well. This case was published in the *British Medical Journal* with Dr Edwards, the anaesthetist, and me as co-authors. It was the first recorded case in Britain of a plastic tube lost in the venous system.[*]

As a teaching registrar, I had two operating lists with Mr Rickham, one with Miss Forshall and one of my own. Since there was a large number of patients on my list, I would try

---

[*] T.E. Udwadia and E. Edwards, 'Plastic Tube Lost in the Venous System', *British Medical Journal*, 1963.

and accommodate as many of them as I could. Once a week, I had to operate at a peripheral hospital where there were no paediatric surgeons. One of these hospitals had an operation table with a plate that read, 'Watson Jones operated on this table'. I felt very pleased to operate on the same table as a great British orthopaedic surgeon.

I had decided to take the London FRCS in May. I sent for the form, filled it, wrote out a cheque, put them in an envelope, addressed it and put it away, planning to post it after a week. One day in April, I got a message from Dr Jackson Rees, the consultant anaesthetist, asking me to post the major cases on my operations list early the next morning as he wanted to leave the theatre at noon sharp. I did so and, during the first surgery, I asked Dr Rees if he was leaving at noon for something important. He said that if he left later, traffic on the M1 would be so heavy that he would not be able to reach London in time for the meeting of the Royal College of Surgeons Council. Suddenly, I realized that I hadn't yet posted my application for the FRCS exam and the deadline was the following day. I told Dr Rees about my problem and, to my consternation, he said that the deadline was not the next day but the same day itself.

He asked if I would be able to give it to him before he left for London. Leaving the closure to my houseman Allan, I rushed home, retrieved the envelope and handed it to Dr Rees in time. Had it not been for this fortunate coincidence, I would not have been able to appear for the London FRCS in May, and probably never would have taken it because I didn't want to continue beyond June at Royal Liverpool.

The London theory exam went well. One question which stumped all the candidates was on the physiology of open-heart surgery. But since I'd worked with Prof. Sen, I knew the answer. I also knew that the English FRCS practicals were very tough and was nervous before the exam. Then, I remembered that Arthur D'Sa, my chief at Wadia, had recommended a swig of brandy to calm down before an exam. So, I poured a small amount into a bottle and put it in my coat pocket. Half an hour before the exam, I drank the brandy and ate a full bar of Cadbury's chocolate to do away with the smell.

I first had the long case. There were two assessors, one quite young and very smartly dressed, and the other elderly, in a worn tweed jacket with an unlit pipe in his hand. After I'd checked the patient, the smartly dressed examiner asked me what my diagnosis was. I said it was a post-nephrectomy arterio-venous fistula. He asked me if I'd ever seen such a case before. I said no, and that, in fact, such a condition should never occur because the artery and the vein are ligated separately and arterio-venous fistula can only occur if the vessels are transfixed with a needle. Having worked with Prof. Sen, I had good knowledge of arterio-venous fistulas. But I could make out that the examiner had found me inadequate during the discussion. The other examiner then got up and said, 'Sonny, I will take you for the short cases.' As we were approaching the patients, he stopped and said, 'Sonny, the more cases you see, the more marks you get. So, let's us be quick in our diagnosis and see as many cases as we can. Have you understood?' I said, 'Yes, sir.' I realized that this man felt that I had not been fairly treated by the first examiner and wanted to help me.

There were two rows of cases, seven cases in each. He started with the front row and most of these were almost spot diagnoses. He would ask, 'What's this?' or he would ask me to palpate a lump and, even as I was giving the diagnosis, he would take me to the next case. I realized that he was rushing me through the cases to make sure that I would finish them all. He then took me to a small room where there were only three patients and said, 'Sonny, select any one. I'll give you five minutes to examine.' The nearest patient had a history of uncontrolled diabetes, bilateral cataract and a dislocated shoulder that was totally pain-free. The bell rang. My five minutes were over. The examiner, without saying anything, looked up at me, waiting for my diagnosis. I said that I couldn't give a proper diagnosis since the man had a neurological condition that resembled—but wasn't—syringomyelia. The examiner then asked me what the cause of the painless shoulder dislocation and the bilateral cataract was. I thought for a moment, then said diabetic neuropathy.

As soon as I said that, I knew I had passed the FRCS. I had never seen any examiner so keen to pass a candidate. I decided that if ever I became an examiner, I would be like him. I came across this examiner once again for the histology slide reading. I said it was a section of a toe, but I didn't know the pathology. He told me to leave it alone as it didn't matter.

When the results were announced at 7 p.m., the first number the porter read out was eleven. I got a shock—my number was twelve and I reasoned that if the first ten had failed, surely both eleven and twelve couldn't have passed. But then, after what seemed to be a very long pause, the porter said, 'Twelve!' That was one of the happiest nights of my life. I phoned Khorshed immediately from the nearest phone booth and could hear her cry with joy.

The next morning, I went to the post office and sent a telegram home, totally bereft of any humility—'Veni, Vidi, Vici, Dublin, Edinburgh, London.' At the hospital, the nurses were all waiting. Once again, I put my thumbs up and they applauded and cheered. They were proud of me as I was to be their registrar.

When I told Mr Rickham that I'd passed, he said that the annual Liverpool Medical Ball was going to be held at the Adelphi Hotel the following day, and as a token of how proud he was of me, he was inviting Khorshed and me. I didn't look at the invitation card he gave me, but when Khorshed and I read it at home, it said, 'Cocktails and Dinner. Dress: Tails and Decorations'. I asked Khorshed what that meant and she said formal attire, and also that since I didn't have a dinner jacket, I'd have to rent one. I refused. I had just passed the FRCS exam the day before and was walking on air. I told her that I'd got a perfectly good suit and that would have to do.

The next day, we got a nurse to babysit the children. I wore my suit, Khorshed wore her beautiful saree and we set off. It was a very pleasant evening and we drove to the Adelphi, Liverpool's most exclusive hotel. To get to the Adelphi's ballroom, you have to climb a flight of stairs to a platform and then walk down another flight. A hall porter stood at the top of the staircase, announcing the invitees. As we stood in the queue, card in hand, Khorshed and I saw the people in the ballroom. There were ladies wearing tiaras and men in tails with their medals—everybody was dressed to the nines.

As we were inching closer to the porter, Khorshed and I looked at each other, looked at my suit and then she shook her head and said, 'No way.' We turned around and went to the reception and Khorshed asked for her stole, making some excuse to the receptionist about forgetting to hand over the formula to the babysitter. We said we'd be back soon but of course we weren't going to.

What were we to do? We couldn't go back home because the babysitter would tell all the nurses that we'd returned very quickly from the ball. So, we drove around Liverpool for a while and when we were hungry, entered a nondescript Chinese restaurant. Everybody there looked astonished to see a pretty young lady in a shimmering gold saree, her hair in a bouffant, having a cheap meal. We took as long as we could over the meal, drove around the city some more and then, when we felt we'd been away for a reasonable time, returned home. The nurse was surprised that we'd come back so soon, but Khorshed said I was tired. I have never lived this incident down and Khorshed has never forgotten to remind me about it at every opportunity. I was and am ashamed that my stupidity and stubbornness deprived Khorshed of her only memorable occasion in the UK.

I decided that since we had not seen anything of England except Liverpool, we should go to the beautiful Lake District for a seven-day holiday. We saw as much as we could, including Wordsworth's house, Windermere. I also felt that some of the smaller, less touristic lakes were beautiful too.

I put in my resignation, much to Mr Rickham's annoyance. Then my parents-in-law came over. Khorshed, the children and all our luggage went to London by train while I drove up in our car. We stayed for a few weeks in London in a hotel opposite Hyde Park. We loved the city, with its beautiful botanical gardens, free art galleries and superb theatre. Then Khorshed's parents and the children left for Bombay while we got ready for our dream trip of Europe in our old Ford.

We had £360 to spend, having already paid for our passage back home by sea in the first week of September. We started from Dover and at Calais, forgetting that I now had to drive on the right side of the road, almost had a collision. We had decided that we would live as cheaply as possible and see as much of Europe as we could. Usually, we would stay in a bed-and-breakfast outside the city we visited—that was much cheaper. We'd have a hearty breakfast and drive off to see the sights. Sometimes, we also stayed at Salvation Army hostels. Those rooms were small but free. On some nights, we even slept in the car. We had the holiday of a lifetime, travelling all over France, Italy, Germany, Switzerland, Austria, Holland and Belgium.

When we returned to London, we found a heap of aerogrammes from Bombay. Something was obviously amiss. We phoned Bombay and learnt that Rushad was very ill with typhoid fever and that we needed to return immediately. We cancelled our steamship tickets and booked ourselves on Air India. We sold the car for £120 and Khorshed spent the money on a silver-plated cutlery set from Mappin and Webb and a Wedgwood dinner set for twelve from Selfridges. Two days later, we flew to Bombay.

8

Returning to Bombay

When I was in Liverpool, I was told that there would be a vacancy at JJ Hospital for the post of an assistant honorary surgeon. Since I was from KEM, I assumed I wouldn't get the job, but applied anyway. Of the fourteen candidates, I was the only one not from JJ and the last to be called. However, Dr Virkar, the dean of JJ and a former KEM man, was overseeing all the proceedings and at one point, he told the committee that whereas the other thirteen candidates, some quite senior, had not published a single paper, I had already published seven. Despite this, I was certain I wouldn't be selected.

Soon after my return, I met Prof. Sen and thanked him for getting me the job at the Royal Liverpool Hospital when I desperately needed one. His answer was typical of him. 'I got you a job?' he asked. 'Do you think I run an employment agency?' Dr Sen never wanted to be seen in a good light; he always wanted to be the big bad boy. He then offered me a full-time job as assistant professor of surgery at KEM on a monthly salary of ₹790.

I thanked him but said I couldn't accept his offer. My colleagues were already earning ten times that in private practice and to make a decent living, I'd have to be dishonest and moonlight, which I would not do. He said in that case he would like me to continue as research fellow in the department of surgery. It would be part-time and allow me to have other hospital attachments, so I could earn an income that would be sufficient for my family. I happily accepted his offer because I knew I would be doing good academic work.

Within two months of my return, I was additionally appointed assistant surgeon at Wadia Children's Hospital. Working there was wonderful. Dr Subhash Dalal, who had returned after three years in the US, was Dr Irani's assistant honorary and Dr R.K. Gandhi and I were Dr Arthur D'Sa's assistant honoraries. Soon, Dr D'Sa retired, Subhash became chief and I became his assistant honorary.

There is a congenital condition called tracheo-oesophageal fistula in which the windpipe is connected to the food pipe. As a result, saliva and fluid from the food pipe and/or stomach can reflux into the airway causing severe, even fatal, lung problems. The connection between the trachea and the oesophagus has to be divided and closed; the oesophagus has to be mobilized and lengthened, and its two ends have to be connected. Operating as such on a newborn is a major undertaking because it has to be done in the chest and is time-consuming. There should be no leak in the anastomosis between the narrow ends of the oesophagus. Even if there is no leak, just the operative procedure is very traumatic for the child.

In the history of Wadia, all the children who'd been operated on for tracheo-oesophageal fistula had died after surgery. So, whenever there was such a surgery, all of us consultants would be present, trying to do our utmost to make the operation a success. At times, there was no nitrous oxide at Wadia and Ramnik Gandhi—who was a paediatric surgeon at KEM—and I would borrow cylinders from KEM. We managed to get two infant incubators and kept the children in them. This was our ICU.

For quite a while, despite everything we did, we failed to save the patients. Finally, when we had our first survival, we felt as if we'd climbed Mt Everest! The conditions we were working in were, by present-day standards, primitive. So was the post-operative care. Our success drove home the importance of the entire staff working as a team for one objective.

At Wadia, I saw several cases of hydrocephalus. In this condition, the outlet of fluid in the brain is blocked and accumulates in the brain itself; distends the soft skull of the newborn child, and the resultant pressure destroys brain tissue. In Liverpool, these children were treated by using a Pudenz valve. But this valve, which had to be imported, cost about ₹20,000 in India, and none of our patients could afford it. It was heartbreaking see them deteriorate. For a long time, I wondered what we could do to overcome this problem. Finally, it dawned on me that perhaps I could use the strong valves in a mother's saphenous vein to treat her child.

I took the saphenous vein of one mother to the department of experimental surgery in KEM. There, I found that hardly any pressure was needed for the fluid to go in the direction of the valve and the valve itself could resist more than 120 mmHg of pressure without letting any fluid go beyond it. I started this procedure on children with hydrocephalus. A plastic tube was inserted into the dilated ventricle and brought through a subcutaneous tunnel. The tube in the neck was attached to the mother's vein which was reversed, with the valve facing the jugular vein so that it prevented blood from going to the brain. I then did a delicate anastomosis (suturing) between the mother's saphenous vein and an opening in the child's small jugular vein. Cerebrospinal fluid from the brain flowed into the venous system, exactly as in the Pudenz valve, ensuring no further brain damage and reducing the hydrocephalus.

In the third week of December 1963, I was surprised to receive a government gazette letter saying that I was appointed as an assistant honorary professor of surgery, Grant Medical College and assistant honorary surgeon at JJ Hospital. Much later, I learnt that Dr Virkar had attached his own note to the selection committee's recommendations saying that, in his opinion, I was by far the most eligible candidate and would bring much-needed academic activity to JJ. So now, I had a foot in three camps—JJ, Wadia and KEM.

Being the junior-most assistant honorary at JJ, I was appointed as honorary surgeon to the minor surgery department. It had two operating tables and around forty to sixty patients a day. Assisting me was Joseph, an efficient OT nurse who had worked in the department for five years. He knew everything that needed to be done and how it had to be done. I am sure that, left to himself, he could have managed the department efficiently.

We had to handle a wide variety of interesting cases. One of them was the simple ganglion. This is a cystic swelling at the wrist with a small communication to the wrist joint. The classic treatment was to hit it with the family Bible, but that didn't always work. Soft ganglions I could rupture and bandage tightly. But although hard ones could be removed surgically, they frequently recurred. I felt that this was because the base of the ganglion, which was in communication with the wrist joint, was always left behind. So, I started excising the cystic swelling and applying carbolic acid to the base of the ganglion in the hope that the acid would destroy the ganglion cells that were responsible for the recurrence. It worked and there were fewer recurrences.*

We did vasectomies by the dozen but on one occasion, after I'd completed one side, I could not find the vas on the other side. I looked for it for forty-five minutes, separating every artery, every vein and the connective tissue. I was afraid that, if I looked any further, I would injure the blood vessels and cause damage to the testis. So, I closed the wound and told the patient to have a semen examination done after four weeks. To my surprise, the report showed no spermatozoa. I looked up the literature and found that there was a condition of agenesis of the vas where the vas does not develop in the foetus. I wasn't aware of this unusual condition and reported it because it carried surgical and medico-legal implications.**

We also saw a large number of labourers who, after hitting their thumbs or fingernails with a hammer, had very painful

---

* T.E. Udwadia, M.M. Omar and A.R. Nazir, 'The "Simple" Ganglion,' *Journal of the Indian Medical Association*, 1974.
** T.E. Udwadia, 'Agenesis of the Vas Deferens—Its Clinical Implications,' *Indian Journal of Medical Sciences*, Vol. 21, No. 3, pp. 185 -188, March 1967.

swellings with blood under their nails, also called a subungual haemotoma. It struck me that since the nail is merely an appendage of the skin, if I could touch the nail with a red-hot pin, it would melt, making a neat hole. The blood could then be squeezed out under local anaesthesia. So, I heated the head end of a pin over a spirit flame till it was red-hot, then touched the nail with it. It would go through the nail like a hot knife through butter and the haematoma would be squeezed out through the hole. The finger would then be tightly bandaged to make sure that fresh blood would not collect under the nail. Thanks to this procedure, the nail was saved, the labourer was totally pain-free and immediately fit for work.

I published papers on all three conditions—ganglions, agenesis of the vas and subungual hematoma.[*] Thanks to my work with Prof. Sen in KEM's department of experimental surgery, my mind was open to new treatment avenues for even minor conditions.

* * *

1964 was the silver jubilee year for the ASI and a conference was to be held in Bombay, at KEM, with Dr R.N. Cooper as the chairman and Prof. P.K Sen as the secretary. Dr Cooper was a good friend of my father's and when I told him that his friend R.N. Cooper was the only surgeon to be twice made president of the ASI, he half-jokingly told me that I'd become ASI president at its golden jubilee. Sadly, he did not live to see his prediction come true.

---

[*] T.E. Udwadia, 'Subungual Haematoma—A Simple and Effective Treatment,' *Journal of the Indian Medical Association*, 1970.

At the 1965 ASI conference, twelve or thirteen surgeons passed a resolution to form a paediatric surgery section. Among the founder members, six were from Wadia and we decided to have a two-day conference of the paediatric section at the hospital the following year. We used the orthopaedic ward as a lecture room, shifting the patients in it to other wards.

There were over 200 registrants for the conference, including several general surgeons and almost every paediatric surgeon in the country. I presented my work on hydrocephalus. To my surprise, Prof. P.K. Sen was in the audience and he congratulated me on my innovation.[*] Two years later, at the International Paediatric Surgery Conference in Liverpool with Prof. Rickham as the chairman, I presented a paper on my work, adding many more cases. It was well-received and the chairman of the scientific committee requested me to write the paper for the *Archives of Disease of Children*. It was published in that journal in 1969.[**] A few years later, Dr Upadhaya, a Delhi-based paediatric surgeon, made a prosthetic valve which was both affordable and functioned longer than the saphenous vein graft. I then stopped doing my procedure and promoted Upadhaya's.

So great was the divide between JJ and KEM, that the JJ surgeons decided not to participate in the conference and persuaded Nair Hospital surgeons to boycott it too. In fact, I was warned that if I attended the conference and presented the two papers that I was scheduled to, I would be dismissed

---

[*] T.E. Udwadia, 'Hydrocephalus in Infancy and Childhood,' *Pediatric Clinics of India*, 1968.

[**] T.E. Udwadia, 'The Treatment of Hydrocephalus Using a Saphenous Vein Graft,' *Archives of Diseases of Children*, 1969.

from JJ as I was still under probation. But I was not willing to be pushed around. As I was also in the department of experimental surgery at KEM, I took an active part in the organization of the conference. However, since surgeons from all over India were coming to the conference, the JJ doctors finally realized that they'd be totally isolated. On the final day, they decided to drop their protest and attended the conference.

Dr Radhakrishnan, the president of India, inaugurated the conference. He gave a most memorable forty-five-minute address in which he combined philosophy, religion and health, and received a standing ovation. No wonder, 5 September, Dr Radhakrishnan's birthday, is celebrated all over the country as Teacher's Day.

Since KEM, JJ and Wadia were all charity hospitals, I wasn't making much money. And because all my father's patients were poor, he'd refer practically all his surgical cases to me at JJ where, of course, they were treated for free. Only once in a while would he get patients who could pay—and that too, not much. I would operate on them at the inexpensive City Clinic, a shoestring operation where the fee was just ₹20 for a bed and medical care. It had one OT and a nurse, the efficient and honest Sister Sheikh, who was the theatre superintendent, matron and administrative officer all rolled into one. Leftover pieces of catgut were stored for the next case, preserved in jars of spirit. When I discussed this with Dr Chaubal who also used to operate there, he said, 'The most important cause of post-operative infection is the surgeon, not the environment.'

Dr Kapasi, the only doctor at City Clinic, was not an MBBS—I think he was qualified in Ayurveda—but he was a competent surgical assistant. He made sure the patients were comfortable and happy and, from him, I learnt that it's not the nature of the medical degree that makes a doctor but the quality of the person. Some of my best residents have not been MBBS doctors.

The very first surgical case my father referred to me at City Clinic was an inguinal hernia. After the procedure, the patient was kept in the hospital for a week—that was the routine for all surgeries in those days—and I saw him every day until his sutures were removed. For all this, I charged him ₹200. But when I told my father about it, he was very angry. He accused me of looting a poor man, and said that when the patient came to me for a check-up, I should give him ₹100 back! From then on, I told my father to write down the fee that I should charge whenever he referred a patient to me.

Apart from my father's referrals, my college friend Chandi Gupta, who had done his MRCP (Member of the Royal College of Physicians) and was Hindustan Lever's physician, referred company employees who needed surgery to me. Some operations I did at City Clinic and some at Bacha's, a higher grade nursing home.

I started my very first consulting room in 1964. A year later, my father persuaded Farokh and me to share a large space in the centre of town with a common waiting room and separate consulting rooms. The location was excellent. I could see the famous Rajabai Clock Tower from my consulting room and, although there was no air-conditioning, there was a nice, cool breeze in the evenings. My father bought me an electric sterilizer and some basic surgical instruments for minor surgeries—which I have till today.

The waiting room was soon full of Farokh's patients, but hardly anyone came to see me. Not only did no GP send me a patient, neither did a single consulting physician. I was busy from morning till evening at three charity hospitals, but I had no private practice to call my own. But I refused to budge; I'd vowed never to split fees.

* * *

From 1966, Dr O.P. Kapoor and Dr K.M. Mody—both JJ physicians who used to refer their surgical work to my JJ unit—started referring work to me at my consulting room.

For my first year of private practice, Joseph, the minor surgery assistant from JJ, was the secretary and receptionist. Whenever there was a chance to do minor surgery, I would do it in my consulting room with Joseph's assistance. But most of the time, Joseph would sit alone in the waiting room and I would sit alone in the consulting room, keeping myself busy writing surgical articles as well as articles for pharmaceutical companies for their informative booklets. Since I was paid per page, I'd try and make the article as long as possible. The second year, I read surgical books as well as books from my library. But, by the third year, I was so fed up that I couldn't read and sat around feeling extremely frustrated. My frustration was largely mitigated by the fact that I was doing good work at JJ, Wadia and KEM.

I tried to get an attachment to the Parsee General Hospital. However, the superintendent, Dr H.S. Mehta, kept telling me that he would take me in as a consultant, but after some time. Fortunately, Khorshed's parents had gifted her a flower shop and that was a slow but steady source of income for the family.

After a year, Joseph left for a job in Dubai and I got a new secretary, Ms Mani Framroze. One day, in April 1967, Mani came to my consulting room looking very excited and said that a patient had come to consult me! It wasn't a patient, but a school friend of mine, Salim Currim, an insurance agent who wanted me to buy a life insurance policy. I told Salim I was sorry, but I couldn't oblige him since I couldn't afford the premiums. He was amazed that despite my qualifications and teaching hospital attachments, I had no practice worth the name. But I promised him that once I could, I'd buy life insurance only from him. Which I eventually did.

A few weeks later, I got a call from a lady saying that she was the secretary of Kenneth Bond, the consultant surgeon at Breach Candy Hospital, and that she wanted to speak to Dr Udwadia. I told her that she had the wrong Dr Udwadia, and that she must want my brother who was attached as a physician to Breach Candy Hospital. She said no, she did not want physician Udwadia but surgeon Udwadia. She asked if I would be free to see Mr Bond at Breach Candy at 3 p.m. the following afternoon. I was overjoyed—here was an opportunity to go to Breach Candy Hospital which I'd last entered ten years earlier as Dr Baliga's assistant. I wanted to tell her that I'd be pleased to see Mr Bond even at 3 a.m.!

On the dot of three the next day, I met Mr Bond, a tall, erect, affable Englishman in a white coat that British army officers used to wear and white trousers. Peering at me through half-rim glasses, he asked if I'd be willing to be his locum as he was going out of India for his holiday. I told him I would be happy to be his locum, expecting that he would be away for two to three weeks. But it turned out that he was going to be away much longer—he travelled only by sea and planned to be in England for three to four months. He was leaving on 2 May and requested that I start from the first.

That was wonderful from my point of view. The longer I was at Breach Candy, the happier I would be. I wondered, though, why he had selected me to be his locum—we hadn't met each other before. One good thing leads to another. A few days later, Dr H.S. Mehta, the Parsee General Hospital superintendent, sent me a letter of appointment as assistant honorary surgeon, also from 1 May 1967!

At 2 p.m. on 1 May, Breach Candy Hospital called me: an English sailor on a ship in harbour had been admitted with a severe facial injury that needed surgery. At that time, the Bombay docks were exceedingly active and all sailors, by mandate, had to be brought to Breach Candy Hospital for treatment. It was part of the agreement on which the hospital was founded.

I was happy and excited at the news—this would be my very first operation at Breach Candy. I was in such a state that immediately after I'd scrubbed and worn my gown, I started walking towards the operation table. Sister Roberts, the theatre superintendent (most of the senior nurses were English in those days) who was going to assist me, said, 'Mr Udwadia, in this hospital, we usually wear gloves when we operate!' Embarrassed, I pulled on my gloves. The sailor's injuries, which included a badly damaged nose, required careful work. When I finished after two hours, Sister Roberts—somewhat hesitantly, I felt—said, 'This is a good job.' But I got on well with Sister Roberts. She was a very fair, firm and competent theatre assistant. She usually scrubbed with me when I was operating.

On my way to Mr Bond's consulting room through the patient waiting area, I met Farokh on his way to his own consulting room. He seemed annoyed to see me and asked what I was doing at Breach Candy. 'I am working here as Mr Bond's locum,' I replied and added, 'for five months' to rub it in. 'Why was I not informed?' he asked. 'Obviously because Mr Bond did not feel that you were required to be informed,' I answered.

While I was a locum at Breach Candy, I was not upset that my brother, the consulting physician, did not refer me a single case because the two hospital outpatient doctors, Dr M. Meraney and Dr B. Meherhomji, referred all surgical cases to me. In addition, I was kept busy in the emergency room of the hospital. At that time, there were few hospitals in the area and Breach Candy catered to many emergencies from Colaba to way beyond Juhu. I happily attended to them at least three or four nights every week.

I had a very satisfying routine those days: outpatients and operations once a week at Parsee General, ward rounds and bedside clinics for students at JJ on the three days I wasn't operating, finishing my experiments at KEM and also attending Wadia Children's Hospital since the two hospitals were opposite each other. Additionally, on my two operation days at JJ, I would work in the OT till about 3 p.m., then go to Breach Candy Hospital for a clinic or to operate on patients. From there, I went to my consulting room and saw patients till late in the evening. Working long hours was most satisfying.

By this time, I'd found out how I got a toehold in Breach Candy Hospital. Mr Bond's secretary, Fareeda Currim, was my school friend Salim's wife. Fareeda, an extremely efficient lady, managed everything for Mr Bond, except operating—she booked his theatre, arranged his consultation and operations lists, collected his fees and kept in touch with all his patients. In short, she ran Mr Bond's show. Apparently, Mrs Currim had had a disagreement with Mr Bond's previous locum over a financial matter. And just a few days before they had to decide who would be his replacement, Salim had spoken about me and my problems to Fareeda. Since I was a surgeon at JJ as well as at Wadia, Fareeda reckoned that I must be doing a lot of surgeries and suggested me to Mr Bond.

I expected that I'd no longer be at Breach Candy once Mr Bond came back. But two days after he returned to Bombay, he sent for me and asked if I would be ready to work with him permanently. He was essentially a colorectal surgeon so he could do with help in general surgery. This was again because of Fareeda, who'd told her boss that all my patients were happy with me and that I was more interested in work than in money.

Kenneth Bond had trained at St Mark's Hospital, a famous London colorectal centre and was about to be appointed as a consultant there when the Second World War broke out. He then joined the medical corps in the army. But after the war, he was no longer in the running at St Mark's, so he decided that he would practise in Bombay. Breach Candy Hospital was being set up and he was requested to take charge as the consultant surgeon. In those days, the 'British is better' attitude still prevailed among many Indians and they preferred to go to an Englishman for surgery.

Thanks to my association with Mr Bond, I got to meet a number of well-known Indian families. And when he retired two years later, his patients continued to come to me at Breach Candy. Getting into Breach Candy Hospital was a great boost for me and my practice. When Mr Bond retired, my brother, who was by then well-installed at Breach Candy Hospital and was friendly with the chairman and all the trustees, had Dr K.N.

Dastoor appointed in Mr Bond's place. Dr K.N. Dastoor was senior and a very good surgeon and though I had been working at Breach Candy Hospital for three years, I readily accepted the correctness of Dr Dastoor's appointment.

There was a friend and colleague of mine at JJ Hospital, Dr H.R. Manchanda, who also had several of his patients at Breach Candy Hospital. He knew several trustees at Breach Candy Hospital and ensured that while Dr Dastoor was to use Mr Bond's consulting room, both Dr Manchanda and I would rotate for all emergencies at Breach Candy with Dr Dastoor—each of us would be on call for a week. It was kind of Dr Manchanda to include me with him, and that is how I got a formal appointment to Breach Candy. Dr Manchanda and I worked side by side, supporting each other through hospital politics, as very good friends and colleagues, for the next fifty-four years.

In the meanwhile, my practice continued to grow at Parsee General Hospital although initially I had some very traumatic experiences there. In the beginning, the only patients I had were on the ground-floor general ward who were admitted from my outpatient clinic. An occasional patient would be referred to me by Dr K.M. Mody who was also attached to Parsee General Hospital, as well as Dr C. Wadia and Dr D.H. Gamadia.

On one occasion, while I was examining the only patient I had at that time in the free ward, my brother Farokh trooped in with his retinue of housemen and nurses to a patient two beds away and told his registrar in his loud, commanding voice to refer this patient to Dr Fardun Soonawala for surgery. That was heard by the entire ground-floor ward of Parsee General Hospital and I am sure every patient there must have been wondering that, if my brother did not refer even a free patient to me, I could not be all that good as a surgeon. I had no grouse with the Soonawala brothers; they always had my respect and affection. I admired the brotherly bond they shared. I survived several such humiliations and ultimately, by giving full care, attention and satisfaction to free patients, my practice slowly grew and bloomed at Parsee General Hospital.

From 1970, my clinical and surgical work mushroomed beyond my wildest expectations. With attachments at JJ, Breach Candy, Parsee General and other hospitals, as well as being a consultant to the armed forces and the central railways, I was kept really busy. During this time, I operated on a large number of Arab patients, thanks to Dr K.M. Mody and Dr O.P. Kapoor, both of whom referred their Arab surgical patients to me. Although most Bombay doctors gave preferential treatment to Arabs, I made no distinction between my patients, irrespective of whether they were locals or foreigners. My Arab patrons weren't allowed to jump the queue and were charged the same fees as Indian patients. While Mani was upset because she felt that this approach would deter them, the Arabs saw that I was treating them fairly and my practice grew by word of mouth. Having said that, whereas I'd always have Indian patients, the Arabs could go as suddenly as they had appeared.

Once, Dr Mody referred a fairly well-built Arab lady with a swelling in her cheek to me. Two surgeons had already told her that she required major plastic surgery, possibly through her mouth, under general anaesthesia. She was told that her nerve could be injured and she would need to be in hospital for at least five days. What she actually had was a big, uninfected sebaceous cyst which could be excised as an OPD procedure, using local anaesthesia. I explained this to her and gave a note to Dr Mody. She left my office in a huff and berated Dr Mody for sending her to a stupid doctor who said that this major surgery could be done as an OPD case!

However, Dr Mody persuaded her to return to me, and after the procedure was over, she realized that I'd saved her from being taken for a ride. On her last visit, she told me that she was the owner of the Ambassador, a large hotel in Dubai, and scolded me for wearing an Indian watch whereas both she and Dr Mody wore Rolexes. Then she removed her watch, put it on my table and asked me to wear it. I refused. Fuming, she took her Rolex and left. In less than ten minutes, Dr Mody rang me up saying that this lady was now angry with him because I hadn't accepted her watch. 'Please accept her watch,' he requested, 'she's an important patient who refers many people to me.' The next day, the lady came to my consulting room before I arrived, handed over the Rolex to my secretary and asked her to give it to me. Of course, I never wore it, but it's now with my son Rushad who collects watches.

After I finished my stint in minor surgery, I could have been posted in any of the six units at JJ Hospital. Major Irani, with whom I was working at Wadia Children's Hospital, went to the dean, Dr Virkar, and told him, 'I want Udwadia in my unit.' Major Irani never made requests; he only issued statements. Thanks to him, I could grow at JJ because he gave me a free hand.

During the 1970s and 1980s, a tremendous amount of surgical work was being done at JJ. Major Irani would do one case at 10 a.m. on the dot. At JJ, each unit had a chief and two assistant honorary surgeons. I was blessed to have Dr Rasik Patel as my unit's senior assistant honorary. Neatly suited, trim and small-made, Rasik was an outstanding surgeon. Moreover, he was an outstanding human being, ethical and friendly. When I first started operating there, he welcomed me by telling me that I could take my pick from the operation list. He had only one request: he had been doing Saturday emergencies for over twelve years and requested me to take over. I readily agreed and continued to do so for the next twelve years, which meant no socializing or alcohol on Saturdays for that period of time. I hardly drink, but alcohol and surgery never mix. On our OT days, Rasik and I would be operating from morning to late afternoon at JJ. If the registrar was doing a major case, it would be under our direct supervision. All three operation tables were in constant use throughout the operating list. The work in our unit was exceedingly heavy because we had a reputation for good work in the hospital and got a lot of referrals. Further, the registrars were getting good work and they realized that they could get more work if they scouted the medical wards for surgical cases to be referred to our unit.

In 1969, the management of the Jerbai Wadia Children's Hospital drew my attention to the fact that I was a paediatric surgeon at the Wadia Children's Hospital, but was doing general surgery for all age groups in other hospitals, which was unfair to paediatric surgeons. The other paediatric surgeons at Wadia Hospital were doing pure paediatric surgery. I agreed with this viewpoint and left a piece of my heart behind when I resigned from Wadia on a matter of principle. But I was retained on the consulting staff as research paediatric surgeon.

The rule for attachments in those days was that no doctor could be at more than one teaching hospital at a time. JJ Hospital had an objection to my being at two. As JJ was the far more important attachment, I told Prof. Sen I would resign from the KEM experimental surgery department. As always, he

refused to accept my resignation and came up with a solution—
he suggested that I do my PhD. As a research student at KEM,
I could therefore continue working at both teaching hospitals.

As I mentioned earlier, Prof. Sen's burning ambition was to
improve myocardial revascularization in patients with coronary
artery disease. He came up with a brilliant new concept which
he wanted me to work on as my PhD thesis. It was to study
the anatomy of the reptilian heart and see if we could replicate
this in the human heart to improve myocardial vascularization.
To do that, I had to first study the anatomy of a snake's heart.
We chose the Russell's viper since the Haffkine Institute across
the road was manufacturing an antidote to this snake's venom.
They had plenty of them, and were ready to give them to us.

On our first visit to Haffkine, I was given a gunny bag
containing a Russell's viper whose venom glands had been
removed. And although nembutal had also been injected into
its abdominal cavity so that it would be unconscious for three
hours, the snake continued to wriggle a little. Prof. Sen and I
had driven to Haffkine in my small car. When we returned to
my vehicle, I gave Prof. Sen the gunny bag so that I could drive.
He immediately returned the bag to me, professing a sudden
interest in my car: he'd never driven a small car and wanted to
drive mine. I'm sure, though, that the real reason was that he
was too scared to hold the gunny bag!

By the time we reached KEM, the snake was totally
immobile. We put it on a tray and opened its thorax to study its
heart. The Russell's viper's heart had just one thin, microscopic
coronary vessel running on the myocardium. When we slit its
heart open, there were deep narrow crevices—inlets—into the
myocardium. The snake's heart was being supplied with blood
by these minute inlets into the myocardium so there was no

need for coronary circulation. The blood flow was from within the heart chamber to the myocardium. This gave us a strong insight into what we could do to replicate the snake's heart in cases requiring increased blood flow to the myocardium. To work out the details of my research, I spent two weeks studying snake hearts, and comparing them to the hearts of dogs.

My first step was to tie off a dog's major coronary artery; see the area being affected by the lack of blood and then map it by outlining the infarcted area with interrupted black silk stitches. Then, in that area, I would create multiple channels through the full thickness of the dog myocardium, so that blood from the heart cavity could enter these channels and supply the heart muscle. I tried various ways of creating these channels, first with a venipuncture needle which was less than 1 mm in thickness, then with one of 1 mm, and then with other channel-making instruments similar to cork borers used by wine tasters. I then closed the animal's chest cavity and kept the dog in the kennel for six to eight weeks. Weekly EEG recording were done. After the six-to-eight-week period, the dog's chest was reopened and the entire part of the myocardium which had been devascularized and then revascularized using various methods was sent to Dr S. Kinare, the surgical histopathologist, to see if the channels created were still open and if circulation in the myocardium was being restored. When the preparation was ready, that is, the slides were stained, Dr Kinare would explain to me which channels remained open with red blood cells and which areas of the myocardium were free of infarction.

Since a large number of experiments were required before we could substantiate our hypothesis, I used different types of boring instruments, varied the numbers and sizes of the channels, and varied the times between creating the infarct and making the channels. With several permutations and combinations, multiple subsets of the study were carried out. Each subset was discussed between Prof. Sen, Dr Kinare and me.

The study went on for over three years, from 1964 to 1967. After we felt that there was enough evidence to prove that we were able to create revascularization, we published our findings in the *Journal of Cardiovascular Surgery*.[*] That created a fair amount of interest and we continued our work and published a second paper.[**] But despite the fact that the work had been accepted by an international journal, my thesis was debunked as absurd and rejected. I did not get my PhD. To add insult to injury, Prof. Sen was demoted as a guide for PhD students.

When I apologized to Dr Sen for being a party to his demotion, he told me calmly, 'Don't be sorry. Success is not a destination; success is a journey. You and I have journeyed together for four happy years, doing work which we felt was correct and got positive results.'

There is another side to this incident. Thirty years later, long after Prof. Sen had passed away, our procedure, now using CO_2 lasers, has become an accepted method of myocardial revascularization. Prof. Sen was thirty years ahead of his time. Whenever I read new articles on this method of myocardial revascularization, I get great joy and pride in seeing that the very first reference in every article is Sen, Udwadia and Kinare.

---

[*] P.K. Sen, T.E. Udwadia, S.G. Kinare and G.B. Parulkar, 'Transmyocardial Acupuncture,' *Journal of Thoracic and Cardiovascular Surgery*, 1965.

[**] P.K. Sen, T. Daulatram, T.E. Udwadia and G.B. Parulkar, 'Revascularisation by Transmyocardial Acupuncture', *Journal of Thoracic and Cardiovascular Surgery*, 1968.

After my PhD attempt, I did not expect to work any longer at KEM. However, Prof. Sen said that I was to consider myself as a permanent member of its experimental surgery department and should join its heart transplant project. He had already transplanted a dog's heart into the neck of a dog and kept it pumping for a few days. He was working on doing a human heart transplant.

To my joy, I was asked to pair up with Sharad Pandey, my old houseman with Prof. Sen and now an assistant professor in the department of cardiac surgery. Sharad and I worked on the donor side while Prof. Sen and Dr G.B. Parulkar worked on the recipient side. They would remove the heart from the dog which was going to receive a heart, while we would remove the donor dog's heart. I know that to all animal lovers—indeed, to any sensible person, including me—this was a terribly cruel method of learning how to do heart transplants, but at that time, it was the only way we could learn. (In fact, all over the world, every transplant programme—whether for the heart, liver, kidney or any other major organ—is dependent on dogs.)

The plan was to operate simultaneously on two tables near each other. The dogs would be anaesthetized at the same time. Usually, Prof. Sen and Parulkar would remove the dog's heart before we would and Sen would fret and get irritable as he waited.

Finally, Prof. Sen decided it was time to document the entire experimental procedure. At that time, we only had a 16 mm movie camera that belonged to Dr D.K. Karanjiawala, who had been my assistant chief when I was a houseman at KEM, ten years ago. He stood on a high stool so that he could zoom in on both procedures.

For once, Sharad and I completed our procedure at exactly the same moment that Prof. Sen and Parulkar completed theirs. The beating donor heart was put on a stainless steel tray and Sharad started taking it to the other team, 8–10 feet away. Then, horror of horrors, the smooth, shining, fresh beating heart slithered out of the tray and fell on the floor with Dr Karanjiawala dutifully recording everything, including this mishap. Sharad immediately picked up the heart but it slipped through his fingers. After he finally got a secure hold on it, he put it back on the tray, washed it in saline and handed it to Prof. Sen and Parulkar. To his dying day, Prof. Sen believed that Sharad and I had done this intentionally so that it could be recorded on film!

On the day the first human heart transplant in India was scheduled, Prof. Sen firmly instructed me not to be anywhere near KEM. Plenty of photographs were going to be taken and if I was in any picture, my position at JJ Hospital would be in jeopardy.

On 16 February 1968, Prof. Sen and the KEM team performed the first Indian human heart transplant. It was the world's sixth such transplant and only three doctors before Prof. Sen had accomplished this feat. The KEM team did so on a shoestring budget, and by overcoming great odds.

Prof. Sen sent me a letter, typed on the same rickety Remington machine that his testimonial for me had been prepared a few years earlier, saying that while he regretted that we had lost the patient of India's first heart transplant, he commended the tremendous team spirit and the loyalty of everyone in the department. He went on to say that he appreciated my contribution and stressed that I would always be a part of KEM's surgery department. I still treasure that letter.

After a second heart transplant shortly thereafter—the patient lived for a few hours—I recalled another saying, 'The measure of success is not in the achievements attained, but in the obstacles overcome in trying to succeed.' On his table, Prof. Sen had a plaque which read, 'They reach too low who reach for the stars.' This one sentence summarizes his life and his vast contributions to surgery. His disciples, no matter what professional heights they reached, always looked up to him as their guru.

9

Laparoscopy

Whenever people tell me that I did the first laparoscopic cholecystectomy (removal of the gall bladder) in the developing world, I say, 'No, it was not done by me. It was done with the surgical team of Ward 19A at the JJ Hospital, Bombay, supported by the anaesthesia team, the nurses and the ward staff.' Like many events in my surgical career, my introduction to laparoscopy was purely by accident.

In December 1971, I was waiting outside the OT at Breach Candy Hospital, about to go into surgery. Normally, the anaesthetist, Dr Gulab Bhagat, would always be there before me, but on this occasion, he was delayed. Fidgeting, I peeped into the adjacent theatre and saw Dr Nergesh Motashaw conducting a procedure with one eye to a telescope. I asked her what she was doing and she replied that she was doing a laparoscopy. I had never heard that word before. I asked what laparoscopy was and she asked me to take a look. I scrubbed and put my eye to the telescope. I was flabbergasted by what I saw. The entire pelvis was illuminated, with perfect anatomy, colouring and presentation. I requested Nergesh if she could reverse the table tilt. She readily agreed and when the head end was raised, I saw the liver, stomach, duodenum, gall bladder, spleen, colon, bowels, diaphragm, omentum and the entire abdominal anatomy, just as I would have seen during an open surgery. Moreover, the view was complete with magnification, perfect light and vision! It immediately struck me that this was the ideal method of diagnosing patients who came with abdominal symptoms. I have always thanked Dr Bhagat for coming late that day because that opened a new vision for me.

After getting the details of the equipment, I wrote to Karl Storz, the equipment manufacturer in Germany. In those days, the import duty for medical equipment was so prohibitive that it was cheaper for Khorshed and me to go to Germany, buy the equipment and bring it back ourselves.

In February 1972, Khorshed and I drove from Frankfurt to Tuttlingen in a red Japanese car—the cheapest and smallest car we could rent. When we arrived, we were shown up to the office of Mr Karl Storz—big-built, six-foot-four and stern-looking. Since, at that time, no surgeon was using a laparoscope, he took it upon himself to show me his equipment. He had set out the entire range required for diagnostic laparoscopy and explained the workings of the first and the simplest instrument, the Veress needle.

Like any true Indian, the first question I asked him was how much it cost. When he told me, I started haggling. 'It's too much for a simple needle!' I told him. 'Surely, you can reduce the price?'

Storz wouldn't budge. 'Professor Udwadia, fixed price . . . always at Storz,' he replied curtly. And so it went on. With every new piece of equipment that he showed me, I would ask the price and request a reduction, and he would say the same thing, 'Fixed price … always at Storz.' He was getting increasingly irritated, and when we finally came to the telescope, he snapped, 'If you want it, you pay for it!'

Presently, it was time for lunch. Probably feeling that I didn't have much money, he offered to take us out for a meal at a nearby restaurant.

As we were walking through the parking area, he stopped in front of my small red car and shouted, 'This is not possible, this cannot happen in Germany! A Japaneeeese car in Germany!' I said it was the only car I could afford to hire. He looked at me as though I was something the cat had dragged in. During lunch, he spoke only to Khorshed.

On the walk back, he told me, 'You, a surgeon, want to buy a laparoscope, when you know nothing about laparoscopy? I will show you some movies made by the gynaecologist Dr Kurt Semm, so that you understand what a laparoscope is and how it is to be used.'

When we got to the office, he said, 'You are fortunate. We have got a new film projector.' At that time, most teaching films were shot on 16 mm film and loading them on projectors was quite a hassle. Since the loading was taking a long time, I walked over to take a look at the projector. When the loading was over, I said in a very harsh, loud voice, 'Mr Karl Storz, this is not possible. This cannot happen in Germany . . . a Japaneeeese projector in Germany!' The projector was a Fuji!

Storz turned red with anger, got up and came to me. As his large frame bore down on my relatively smaller one, it struck me that I wouldn't need the red car to go back to Frankfurt—I would be going back in an ambulance. Suddenly, Storz burst out laughing. He laughed and laughed and between the Japaneeeese car and the Japaneeeese projector, we forged a friendship with him and the entire Storz family that lasted for fifty years. He did not reduce the price of the equipment, though.

Since I was not buying the insufflator, which was the only large instrument, the equipment we purchased could be put into Khorshed's suitcases, secreted between her sarees and dresses. I had no compunction in smuggling the equipment into Bombay because it was going to be used for poor patients in a teaching hospital with no financial return to me.

From the time I bought Storz's equipment in 1972 till 1990, when the JJ surgical team did the developing world's first laparoscopic cholecystectomy, I used laparoscopy only for diagnosis. I would perform these procedures using local anaesthesia without making a large incision on the abdomen—often as an outdoor procedure—to make a straightforward visual diagnosis. I would also, if needed, photograph, document and biopsy the pathology for final diagnosis.

Initially, every surgeon thought that laparoscopy was an exercise in futility, but several honorary physicians from JJ Hospital started referring their gastrointestinal cases to me. The residents were delighted because they were getting into a totally new field of surgery, which possibly had great future significance.

Though this technique was not well-received in large cities because surgeons thought it was a totally inadequate procedure, it was welcomed in small towns and rural areas. From 1975, I started travelling with this equipment to spread the importance of diagnostic laparoscopy to surgeons who had no investigative facilities and could use it as an essential and cost-effective diagnostic tool. In the process, I travelled throughout the country, north to south, east to west. Later, I wrote a paper on 3000 cases of diagnostic laparoscopy that was published in *Surgical Endoscopy.** We showed that even after including the cost of repairs to the laparoscopic hand instruments and new bulbs for the light source, the total expenditure on the equipment, when spread out over 3000 cases, came to less than ₹10 per patient, making this technology easily affordable in a developing country.

When our paper was sent for publication, it was accepted with just one comment: one of the reviewers said that it was not possible to use the same telescope for eighteen years. I explained how a telescope could be used for that length of time and the journal published my response. Every bit of equipment that we purchased in 1972 was in perfect working condition till 1990. Of course, the equipment was handled gently, as if it were a newborn baby, by the unit surgical staff. Shankar, the head OT assistant, cleaned the equipment even more meticulously than I did.

Laparoscopy gave me the benefits and rewards of travelling through small-town India. I went ostensibly to teach, but after coming back from every place I visited—be it a small town, a rural area or a tribal region—I returned humbled and educated and inspired to do even more because I saw what could be achieved in the face of a total lack of facilities. Diagnostic laparoscopy would also help prepare the ground for the avalanche of laparoscopic cholecystectomies that was soon to follow.

---

* T.E. Udwadia, '30 Years of Diagnostic Laparoscopy—An Overview,' *Surgical Endoscopy*, 2004.

By the time the idea of laparoscopically doing a cholecystectomy started to gain traction, I had the advantage of having done both diagnostic laparoscopy on over 2500 patients and having performed several open cholecystectomies over a twenty-seven-year period. This gave us a head start. In theory, all I had to do was combine the two approaches. But of course, in practice, it wasn't that simple.

The first and foremost principle of all surgery is '*Primum Non Nocere*', which means 'Above All Do No Harm'. In the initial days of laparoscopic cholecystectomies, a large number of life-threatening complications were caused by American surgeons who jumped on to the bandwagon without proper training. Finally, they were made to realize that laparoscopic surgery and open surgery—while achieving the same purpose— were very different techniques.

In laparoscopic surgery, a telescope is inserted into the abdomen through a 1 cm incision at the umbilicus, after insufflating gas into the abdominal cavity. A video camera is attached to the eye piece of the telescope which projects the telescopic vision to a TV monitor. Long, insulated instruments—grasping forceps, scissors, hook and needle-holder—are introduced through 3 mm, 5 mm or 10 mm tubes into the abdomen to perform the surgery.

While laparoscopic surgery is easier on the patient in terms of recovery time, it's harder for the surgeon vis-à-vis open surgery. This is due to many reasons. First, the surgeon can only see what the camera shows them. Second, they operate not on the patient, but on an image on a flat screen. This downgrades 3D vision to 2D, leaving out the important aspect of depth. Third, the long instruments used in laparoscopy restrict wrist movements that the surgeon uses for intricate manoeuvres in open-heart surgery. And finally, it's the tips of the long instruments that are in contact with the tissue, not the fingers, and the surgeon cannot feel what they are doing. To overcome these and other difficulties, a surgeon must train outside the OT on models, pelvi-trainers and simulators. To train on patients is criminal. *Primum Non Nocere.*

To practise for our first laparoscopic cholecystectomy, we created our own model called a pelvi-trainer, fashioned out of a plastic box which mimics the abdomen, with foam cut to replicate abdominal organs, matchsticks, cubes of sugar, uncooked rice, cooked rice and overcooked rice. Now, of course, aspiring laparoscopic surgeons can train on far more sophisticated devices, but that wasn't the case back then. To prepare for the operation, the surgical residents and I practised for six weeks on the pelvi-trainer, after clinic hours, to get a sense of the hand-eye coordination, the feel of the instruments and the right amount of pressure needed so as to not damage tissue. We worked late into the night in my spare bedroom using the home television. We studied a video sent by my friend Professor Alfred Cuschieri doing his first laparoscopic cholecystectomy, replaying it dozens of times, checking and rechecking each movement and manoeuvre.

In addition, every night before I fell asleep and every morning when I woke, I would imagine step-by-step how the patient would be draped, how the procedure would be performed from start to finish as well as how and where the connections for gas, cautery, light and suction would be. I even used my car's door handle to practise tying knots.

In mid-May, we felt we were ready. On 24 May 1990, we did a laparoscopic appendectomy, the first laparoscopic procedure done by our unit at JJ. The laparoscopic cholecystectomy was scheduled for a week later. The patient's name was Anubee. She was from Uttar Pradesh, and I still remember the shiny, large gold earrings she wore.

The night before the surgery, I got an intemperate phone call from one of my peers, accusing me of wanting to do experimental surgery on humans just because I'd done experimental surgery on dogs. If anything went wrong, he warned me, I would be in serious trouble.

It didn't help that the patient had had multiple past episodes of pain in the right hypochondrium, and that the sonography showed a subacute cholecystitis with a thickened gall bladder and multiple stones. It wasn't an ideal case for our first laparoscopic cholecystectomy! I spent a restless night.

The morning of the surgery dawned. Dr Deepraj Bhandarkar, my registrar, came home for a quick breakfast. My small Fiat Padmini was stuffed to the gills with equipment and material for the laparoscopy: in the boot, on Deepraj's lap, my lap, on the seat and on the seat next to the driver. We took pretty much everything: the TV, the instruments and the insufflator. Since the small carbon dioxide (CO_2) cylinder that came with the insufflator would not be adequate for the lengthy procedure that we had anticipated, we bought two large cylinders of CO_2 from a soda-water factory and took them in the car as well.

After we double-checked that the patient and family had been given a full explanation—in Hindi—of the operation, and that a detailed, informed consent had been obtained, she was anaesthetized and placed in the lithotomy position so I could stand between her legs and operate. Anaesthesia was administered by Dr (Mrs) Dhond. The operative team consisted of Deepraj as camera operator and first assistant, Dr Pradeep Kaul, the second assistant and me.

I planned to do the procedure in the same way that I did open cholecystectomies. We had decided to make sure that every small bleeder would be coagulated (cauterized) immediately so that blood would not be allowed to collect in the abdominal cavity. This was not only necessary for vision but also to ensure almost no blood loss during the procedure.

Once the abdomen was insufflated (insufflation is where CO_2 is safely and systematically introduced into the abdomen so that the abdominal cavity expands to create a space for safe surgery), the surgery started. I had just begun the dangerous dissection at Calot's triangle (a 4 mm triangle with important structures), which with the advantage of magnification looked much larger during laparoscopic surgery. I had just developed a good plane of dissection when, unexpectedly, the power went out.

All was deadly quiet. I carefully withdrew the hand instruments and the telescope from the abdomen. Intra-abdominal pressure was reduced to make sure there was no respiratory problem. While a power failure in the hospital was not unusual, it was obviously never welcome, and there was just nothing one could do. At that time, there were no generators, so we had to wait in near darkness.

When the power returned thirty-five minutes later, the abdomen was re-insufflated and the hand instruments re-inserted. But just as we were about to clip the cystic artery, we had a new problem. The insufflator stopped functioning and the gas level dropped. In laparoscopy, tubular structures like the cystic artery or cystic duct are occluded by small titanium clips between which the structure can be safely divided.

However, Deepraj had studied the manual and he figured that the power outage had probably blown a fuse of the insufflator. So, mid-operation, we put in a new fuse and got back on track.

We clipped and divided the artery and then dissected the duct from the gall bladder to about 2 cm towards the common bile duct. We clipped and divided the cystic duct but, just as we started dissecting the gallbladder from the liver, the diathermy equipment stopped working. (Diathermy is electrically induced heat that's used to seal a bleeding vessel and therefore a vital part of operative procedures.) The diathermy cable was found to be faulty. Another cable was sterilized and the surgery resumed. This was our third interruption.

The gall bladder was dissected from the liver fossa with diathermy and was now lying free, ready to be removed. There were two sites one could remove the gall bladder from—either the umbilicus or the epigastric region. For the best surgical outcome, I decided to remove the gall bladder from the epigastric region. I dilated the epigastric incision with an open haemostat and the gall bladder was gradually withdrawn from the abdomen.

Even before I could heave a sigh of relief as the gall bladder came out, there was loud cheering and clapping. We were completely rattled. We'd been concentrating so completely on what we were doing that we didn't realize that almost every surgical resident of JJ Hospital was standing behind us in the OT, silently observing the procedure on the television monitor. The cheering lasted for quite some time and I was amazed to see residents from other specialities too. It was so heart-warming.

With three interruptions, the procedure had lasted a little over three hours. I was more exhausted mentally than physically and my eyes were strained from staring intently at the monitor. The patient was kept in the theatre for two hours to make sure that she was completely stable and then sent to the ward. The resident doctors who had come to watch were reluctant to leave the OT complex, talking animatedly and slapping each other on the back.

As I was sitting in the surgeon's room, some of the doctors came in. It was a great achievement for JJ Hospital, they said, and we must immediately inform the press. I was most annoyed. I insisted that under no circumstances would any information be given to any press. This was a surgical procedure and not a circus act to be publicized. In any case, I pointed out, 'One swallow does not a summer make,' and nobody knew what would happen to the next few cases.

I remained in the surgeon's room for a while, thinking about the surgery. Though the residents were elated, I wasn't. I felt pangs of uncertainty and doubt. After a cup of tea, I changed and went to the ward to check on the patient. She was fully awake, seemed completely well and not in any pain. I palpated her abdomen and there was no tenderness. I congratulated the surgical team and thanked them for their support and loyalty.

That night, I lay in bed reliving every minute of the procedure and wondering where we could have improved upon it. I was trying to compare it with my open cholecystectomy and I couldn't help but feel that open was both faster and safer. I kept agonizing over whether I had done the right thing or whether I'd been on an ego trip, performing a procedure that might not have been in the best interests of the patient.

When I came for rounds the next morning, I was mentally prepared to tell the residents that perhaps laparoscopic surgery required a rethink. But the moment I entered the patient's ward, all my doubts were immediately dispelled. The patient was sitting straight up in bed. If she'd had an open cholecystectomy, she would have been on her back with a Ryle's tube in her nostril and in pain. But her face was bright, her gold earrings glinted in the morning light and she seemed to be quite pleased. I asked her how she was and she immediately replied that she was doing well, and wanted to know why I wasn't giving her anything to eat. Her strong, positive reply made me realize that there was nothing wrong with laparoscopic cholecystectomies—we just needed practice to do it better.

I examined her and found the abdomen soft and totally pain-free. She could take a deep breath without any problems; her bowel sounds were normal, her chest—on auscultation—was normal, and she was cheerful and ready to go home! It was then that I felt that laparoscopic surgery had a great future, particularly in a country like India, where daily-wage labourers have to return to work quickly.

Despite her protestations and out of abundant caution, we kept the patient under observation in the ward for a full five days. To our astonishment, by the second post-operative day, she was on a normal diet and fit enough to go home. She was discharged on the fifth day and was instructed to return after three weeks. At follow-up, she was completely fit and informed us that she had started her daily routine the day she went home.

I could not have done the surgery without my very competent team. Dr Deepraj Bhandarkar, especially, was like a rock. He was the perfect assistant—he was a source of confidence and thought on his feet when he realized that the insufflator's fuse had to be replaced. Dr Pradeep Kaul retracted beautifully—no one would have guessed that this was the first time he was retracting with a long instrument inside the abdomen. Indeed, everyone played their part well.

I was glad that I had decided to do the procedure in the lithotomy position, because there were times when I had to put my eye to the telescope to ensure that what I was seeing on the monitor was exactly as it was in the patient's body. And for thirty years, I have maintained the lithotomy position. It was only later that I came to know that a large number of European surgeons do the procedure the same way.

Word got around and we began to get a few referrals for more laparoscopic cholecystectomies. Cases were being lined up not only at JJ, but at all the hospitals that I was attached to by then, including Hinduja, Breach Candy, Parsee General, Cumballa Hill and Masina. Over the next few procedures, we continued to build our confidence, and took both our team and our equipment from hospital to hospital, not only performing the surgeries but also inviting surgeons to see them. The first laparoscopic cholecystectomy to be done in a private hospital in India was at Hinduja Hospital, two weeks later. I had also brought the residents of Hinduja Hospital home to work on the pelvi-trainer and get a sense of the hand-eye coordination so that they were ready to take over from the JJ residents after a few cases. Deepraj had come for the first case at Hinduja and it is a matter of great pride and joy to me that today, he is the head of the laparoscopy section at that hospital.

Despite the success of the procedures, there was no shortage of surgeons ready to do to us what German surgeons had done to Dr Eric Muhe, who had performed the very first laparoscopic cholecystectomy in Germany. His orthodox professors warned him to stop performing this procedure. During one of his operations, a patient suffered a bile duct injury and Dr Muhe's professors had him put on trial for homicide. The next five years of his life were spent in court, on bail or in jail. *In surgery, the truth often starts as blasphemy!* Things could have also gone horribly wrong for us. In Anubee's case, the dissection of Calot's triangle in chronic cholecystitis was difficult and hazardous. To have a disaster in our first case would have surely put an end to future procedures and, very possibly, landed the entire operative team, including me, in legal trouble. Looking back, I'm sure that repeated visualization of the operation, teamwork and the weeks of meticulous training, often far into the night to take care of all eventualities, was the key to our success.

In our initial experiences of the operation, we found it difficult to remove the large stone load from the gall bladder before extracting it through a small incision. The solution was found by Valentina, the OT nurse at Cumballa Hill Hospital, who suggested the use of ovum forceps, an instrument long discarded by gynaecologists. Valentina's simple innovation was safer and quicker than the sophisticated equipment of the time like lithotripters made for the same purpose, and it was duly credited to her.*

There was no reaction from chiefs of other surgical units at JJ, whereas other senior surgeons criticized us—they were convinced that I was performing experimental surgery on humans and, by implication, playing with their lives. And English surgeons wrote in condescending tones in Indian journals, about how 'laparoscopic surgery was inappropriate and inadvisable for developing countries'. Equally sadly, Indian surgeons, too, questioned our ethics in foreign journals,

---

* T.E. Udwadia and R.T. Udwadia, 'The Ovum Forceps—Safe, Efficient "Lithotripter" and Stone Evacuator for Laparoscopic Cholecystectomy,' *Journal of the Society of Endoscopic and Laparoscopic Surgeons of Asia*, 1996.

accusing us of being stooges of the West, and having no understanding of Indian conditions.

Despite repeated successful surgeries and publishing landmark books on laparoscopic cholecystectomy,* major private hospitals in Mumbai, expecting such procedures would die a natural death, did not invest in laparoscopic equipment. I had to transport my instruments from hospital to hospital. It was only in 1992 that mainstream Indian hospitals decided that they would conduct laparoscopic procedures.

Slowly, workshops on laparoscopy began to be held. By today's standards, these workshops were quite basic, but I'm glad to be able to say that the surgeon who had threatened me with grave consequences if anything happened at my first laparoscopic cholecystectomy was the first surgeon to register for the first course at Hinduja. Three other surgeons from neighbouring countries—all three of whom became presidents of their country's laparoscopic societies—also attended this workshop.

But patients were the main propelling force behind the growth of laparoscopic surgery in India. They realized that this was a boon for them. They had no pain, very short hospital stays, minimal medication, no scars and were able to return quickly to family and work. It was they who drove surgeons to learn laparoscopic surgery.

In 1993, thirty-four surgeons formed the Indian Association of Gastrointestinal Endoscopic Surgeons (IAGES) in Mumbai with me as the president. I had become a member of the Society of American Gastrointestinal Endoscopy Surgeons (SAGES) in

---

* T.E. Udwadia, *Laparoscopic Cholecystectomy* (Mumbai: Oxford University Press, 1991).

March 1990, and was keen to model IAGES along similar lines. The Endoscopic and Laparoscopic Surgeons of Asia (ELSA) society was started in 1991. At its conference in Thailand, I was appointed as the president of ELSA for a three-year term.

I was on the faculty of the first laparoscopic workshop in China, held in the military hospital in Shanghai in 1992–93. At that time, I felt that Bombay was a much more modern city than Shanghai. But over subsequent visits, I was amazed at how rapidly Shanghai was developing and it was depressing to see Bombay slip further and further behind.

Laparoscopic surgery grew phenomenally through the last decade of the twentieth century and, by the beginning of the twenty-first century, India was recognized all over the world as an important laparoscopic centre. The very first dedicated laparoscopic surgery unit was created by Dr Pradeep Choubey at the Gangaram Hospital in Delhi in 1996 and is testimony to what a department dedicated to minimal access surgery can achieve. Today, while surgeons in every major city in the country do first-rate laparoscopic surgery, equally hearteningly, such procedures have penetrated small-town and rural India too.

In my book *Laparoscopic Surgery*, published by Oxford University Press in 1991, I wrote in the preface that 'Laparoscopic cholecystectomy may well be the springboard for new endeavours in minimal invasive and minimal access surgery in areas not even dreamt of today, be it resection of the bowel or even of the liver.' Far from being a fanciful prediction, time has proved it a gross understatement. Today, all abdominal surgery can be done laparoscopically.

10

You Win Some,
You Lose Some: Select Cases

Both Khorshed and I are financially naive. For many years, all of our earnings were kept either in our savings account with the Central Bank of India or in its fixed deposits. I had inherited some shares from my father, but I didn't want to ever sell them. We were aware that this was not the wisest way to invest our money, but we were afraid to consult anyone, in case they took advantage of our ignorance and cheated us. Then, one day in 2000, out of the blue, we got a letter from a young man.

However, he wasn't just any young man. Five years earlier, his father, a Mr Kumar, who had cancer of the oesophagus, had been referred to me by two colleagues at Hinduja. The disease was advanced and his first doctor, certain that the prognosis was poor, had advised chemotherapy and radiation.

Kumar and his wife, however, wanted more radical treatment and insisted on surgery. Their children were still young, they explained, and he wanted to continue working as long as possible. I ultimately agreed to operate but did not give the patient false hope, and objectively discussed the possibility of a poor outcome.

At surgery, I first opened his abdomen and extensively mobilized the stomach—separated from surrounding structures—so that I could bring it high up into his chest. Then, I opened the right side of his chest and widely mobilized the lower third oesophageal tumour, carefully cleared the lymph nodes for spread and excised the tumour and part of the stomach. I brought the stomach into the chest and joined it to the upper end of the oesophagus. Appropriate drains were left in the chest and the abdominal incisions were closed.

The histopathology report revealed clear margins, a squamous cell carcinoma with lymph node spread. Before surgery, Hinduja's Tumour Board had discussed post-operation adjuvant therapy, and three weeks after the operation, Kumar was referred to Dr Asha Kapadia, head of oncology at Hinduja, for further management.

For the first two years, he would come to see me every three months. He was doing well and had no difficulty swallowing. He had gained normal weight and was fully active. As he was now essentially the patient of the oncology department, I gradually saw him less and less often. Then, his wife came to me with breast cancer. I operated on her and then referred her to Dr Asha Kapadia for adjuvant therapy.

The letter that we got from the young man brought both good and sad news. Kumar's son—Ashok—wrote that his father had lived for a little more than five happy years after I'd operated on him. He'd not had any further problems all that time. Both the young man and his brother had graduated and were working. They were married and Kumar had been able to dote on a grandchild for a whole year before his death.

Ashok said that he and the other members of the family were eternally grateful for what I had done for his father and that they'd be more than happy to be of any service to me. He himself was a financial consultant, in the business of advising people the best ways of investing their money.

Khorshed and I immediately felt that this letter was a godsend. Ashok would obviously not cheat us. So, we called him over, and revealed information about all our assets. He listened carefully, noted everything down and shortly afterwards, suggested an investment plan that has, ever since, brought us good returns.

Strange indeed are the ways of the world. I would never have imagined that one of my operations—and that too, not a particularly difficult one with god granting a good result—would make Khorshed and me financially secure.

* * *

The boy with the neurofibromas

Early in my private practice, an English lady, a former nurse married to an Indian, brought her two-year-old son to me. Rakesh had a huge tumour in the parotid region, grossly disfiguring his appearance. His mother told me that she had taken her son to the Royal Liverpool Children's Hospital and had been advised by my former chief, Mr Peter Rickham, to consult me when she returned to Bombay.

I explained to Rakesh's mother that her son had a neurofibroma involving the parotid gland. Removing this tumour would very likely—if not almost certainly—result in damage to Rakesh's facial nerve and his face would not remain symmetrical. The facial nerve supplies all the muscles to the face, the cheek, the eyelid, and without nerve supply, the muscles would not function. I also informed her that a malignant neurofibroma is a nasty lesion to have, but she said that Mr Rickham had already told her all this.

At surgery, my first aim was to identify the trunk of the facial nerve before it entered the parotid so that I could trace it through the tumour and try my best to preserve the five branches. The tumour overlapped the ear and it was only after a slow and careful dissection that I was able identify the facial nerve's trunk. The excision of the entire tumour took four hours of identifying and preserving each branch of the facial nerve as it spread out like the finger of a hand through the tumour. I removed the deep part of the parotid piecemeal from under the spread-out nerves to ensure they weren't damaged. I used a magnifying loupe because the nerves were as thin as fine strands of silk. At the end of the operation, a suction drain was left in. There was a slight deficiency in the upper eyelid's movement, but the rest of the face had normal nerve innervation and looked normal.

The histopathology report revealed that the neurofibroma was benign. Rakesh followed up with me at regular intervals. We became very fond of each other. When Rakesh was about eight, a few neurofibromas appeared on his hand and back. They were excised and all were benign. And from then on, he continued to develop them. Though they were all benign, I was worried. There was always a possibility of a neurofibroma turning malignant. But Rakesh grew up, got married and had a son. I even examined the child and told the mother and the grandmother to keep a careful watch on him.

Some years later, Rakesh's mother called me to say that Rakesh had a huge tumour on his back which he hadn't told anyone about. When I saw it, I was aghast: it was a 2 x 2 inch tumour, 1 inch above the level of the skin. It was ulcerated and obviously malignant. A second opinion confirmed that excision had to be done immediately because it would fungate soon. The prognosis was pretty hopeless because it had spread to other organs. I did a very wide en-bloc excision and used a rotation flap to cover the operated area and split thickness graft over the area of rotation.

Rakesh remained gentle and affectionate; his sole interest was in his wife and son. His devoted parents were devastated by the grim prognosis. For a few months, all was well and then Rakesh was readmitted to hospital in a terminal state of disseminated disease. His heartbroken wife and parents stood by his bed as he was sinking. His mother said, 'Tehemton, please do something.' But there was nothing I could do. I called out his name as loudly as I could. His eyelids fluttered and opened and then recognition registered. He gave a gentle smile to his wife, mother, father and me. He called out to me. Then his eyes closed and he passed away.

* * *

The champion jockey

On a hot April Sunday, more than forty years ago, I was lying down after lunch and drowsily trying to read the newspaper, when I got a phone call saying that a jockey, Karl Umrigar, had fallen off his horse and had been severely injured. I left for Breach Candy Hospital immediately.

I was aghast when I saw the young, handsome jockey, still in riding clothes, smeared with mud, semi-conscious, totally blue and gasping for breath. Frothy blood was gushing out of his nose and mouth. It was obvious that his lungs had been severely injured—his own horse had trampled on him.

The surgical resident told me that he was waiting for a portable chest X-ray. But if nothing was done immediately, Karl was certain to drown in his own blood and die in a few minutes. I cleaned his face and neck as best as I could and, after wearing gloves, quickly performed a tracheostomy. When the blade cut his skin, the blood was not blue but black—he was totally deoxygenated. Through the tracheostomy tube, I sucked out a large amount of blood which had accumulated in his bronchial tree. With that, his breathing improved, but I knew I could not keep up high-pressure suction in his trachea and bronchial cavity for very long because that would prevent air from going in. So, I immediately inserted a low-pressure suction and started ventilation with an Ambu bag.

As soon as he was propped up in the ICU, his colour improved and his heart rate came down. A portable chest X-ray revealed that large parts of his lungs were opaque. I immediately called Dr K.N. Dastoor, a very experienced thoracic surgeon, and requested him to take over the case. Dr Dastoor arrived but said that since the case was admitted under me and I had initiated the essential primary treatment, I should continue the case with him.

Dr Dastoor felt that the bleeding was not going to stop and decided to do a thoracotomy, with me assisting him. We found large areas of lung pulped and bleeding, and Dr Dastoor did segmental and localized resection where necessary. The young jockey was sent back to the ICU on a ventilator.

The bleeding reduced considerably after surgery. Maintaining him required expert intensivist care because the poly trauma had caused severe cardiac and metabolic changes. After a few days, Dr Dastoor thought that it might be worth putting him on the ECMO or Extracorporeal Membrane Oxygenation. This method had been first used just seven years earlier and was considered semi-experimental. The process entailed pumping blood from the patient's vein to drip slowly over a special membrane, while oxygen and air were pumped across the membrane in opposite directions. This, in theory, would rest the lung and give the injured areas a chance to heal and stop the bleeding.

The ECMO at that time was large and bulky with a primitive pressure pump. Venous-to-venous ECMO was carried out. Even though the ECMO's efficacy was not really established at that point, we were convinced that it was our only chance. Karl was a great fighter and gave hope and strength to all of us who were looking after him. His fans camped on the pavement outside the hospital, lined up to donate blood for him and prayed for his recovery. My father-in-law, a racehorse owner, knew his parents.

These days, the ECMO is a small, elegant and portable machine. If that accident had happened today, Karl could have been maintained on it, had a bilateral lung transplant and continued to remain a champion jockey. But in 1979, he slowly slipped away, dying on the eighteenth day of his admission. He was eighteen years old.

Outside medical circles, it is not often appreciated or understood that in such situations, there is always a second victim. The first, obviously, is the patient. The second is the surgeon. For a long time after, I would wake up with a jolt in the middle of the night after seeing this boy in my dreams, the bright colours of his jockey uniform, his handsome face and the bubbles of blood spouting from his nose and mouth. A few months after his death, his parents, with grace and magnanimity, came home with an exquisite gift that still has pride of place in my house. My throat choked with tears and I could not even bring myself to thank them.

* * *

God grants miracles to those who deserve them

In 1986, friends convinced Khorshed and me to purchase an apartment in Pune since prices there were rapidly rising. So, one Sunday, we went to the home of a Pune builder named Ramesh Thakkar and, over lunch, met his wife Mala and their two children, a daughter and a strapping fourteen-year-old boy named Govind. Thakkar then took us to the property. We liked it and completed the deal straightaway. From then on, we would drive to Pune every few months to see the apartment and have lunch with Thakkar and his family. We became good friends.

One evening in 1990, Ramesh called from Pune to say that Govind, now eighteen, had been severely injured in a motorcycle accident. He'd been in a Pune hospital for more than a week and his condition was rapidly deteriorating. Ramesh requested me to take over the case. I said I could only do so if Govind was in Bombay. Ramesh immediately hired an ambulance and brought his son to Breach Candy Hospital.

Govind's injuries were so extensive that I could examine him properly only under anaesthesia in the OT. As he was being wheeled there, he looked at me anxiously. Putting on a cheerful face, I tugged his long, thick black hair and said, 'Champ, we will get you well.' His eyes closed with relief.

Govind had a ghastly 'degloving' injury of the right inferior extremity extending from the hip, the gluteal region, the perineal region and the entire circumference of the thigh down to the lower third of it. The whole degloved flap had been placed back into position in Pune and sutured. He had had a colostomy to prevent faecal contamination of the exposed gluteal and perianal area. He was heading towards septicemic shock.

A 'degloving' injury is a circumferential injury of an extremity where the entire flap of skin and deeper tissue is torn down like a glove being removed. After the accident, Govind had been lying for hours with the deep tissues of his thigh and hip in contact with a filthy under-construction road before a passing friend took him to a Pune hospital.

In the OT, my worst fears were confirmed: gas gangrene had developed. I cleaned the wound meticulously and excised the obvious gangrenous tissue. We pumped anti-gas gangrene serum into him and arranged for hyperbaric oxygen therapy. In this therapy, the patient is placed in an airtight chamber containing oxygen at a high pressure. The oxygen is forced into the contaminated tissues to destroy the gas gangrene organisms—they require an oxygen-free environment to grow.

Normally patients undergo hyperbaric oxygen therapy once a day, but since Govind had had extensive gas gangrene for some time, I organized for him to have two sittings. After he came back from his first visit to the hyperbaric centre, his wound was cleaned in the OT; all the dead tissue was excised and that night, he went to the centre for the second time, and his wounds were dressed again.

Govind stoically and without complaint undertook the two daily trips over ten days in a bumpy ambulance. He also had a fractured pubis so I immediately requested Dr Dholakia, the head of orthopaedics at KEM and also at Breach Candy, to examine him. Seeing the extent of the injury and the deep-seated infection with gas gangrene, Dr Dholakia said Govind wouldn't survive if he didn't have a hindquarter amputation.

A hindquarter amputation is one of the most drastic procedures in surgery. The entire limb with the hip is removed, leaving not even a butt on which any prosthetic could be used or applied. Dr Dholakia had been my teacher, but I couldn't agree with him. 'Sir,' I told him, '. . . he's young and strong. I think he'd prefer to die than have a hindquarter amputation. Please give me two to three days to see if I can reverse the infection.'

After writing 'advised hindquarter amputation' on the notes, Dholakia left the onus on me. Each dressing after the hyperbaric therapy would take well over an hour. The entire degloved area which had lost its blood supply got gangrenous and I had to gradually excise it right up to its base at the knee. The entire hip, gluteal region and thigh were now exposed.

Govind had a ruptured bladder which the urologist Dr Kamath attended to. I also called Dr Keshwani, a plastic surgeon, to take a look at Govind's extensive raw area. But nothing could be done until the infection cleared completely.

After four days of hyperbaric oxygen therapy, Govind's wounds showed some improvement. But when I requested Dr Dholakia to see him again, he still felt that a hindquarter amputation was necessary. I pleaded with him for four more days.

Govind was the most compliant and co-operative patient imaginable. The nurses and resident staff immediately took to this handsome lad who smiled through all that he was going through and they did all they could. Then, what I was dreading most happened: the sciatic nerve, which supplies the inferior extremity, was trapped in the gangrenous muscle, a part of it turned black and started showing bubbles of gas gangrene. I had to excise 4 inches of it along with the surrounding gangrenous muscle. It broke my heart, but I had no option.

Two months earlier, at a laparoscopy workshop that I'd held in Nairobi, I learnt from a surgeon who was a Sanskrit scholar that Sushruta had recommended ghee and honey dressings for non-healing, infected wounds. I had tried it at JJ and was gratified with the results.[*] Govind was the first patient outside JJ to have ghee and honey dressings. And once the infection had cleared, Dr Keshwani spent hours grafting the entire area bit by bit. The interesting thing is that every doctor and nurse took it upon themselves as a mission to try and salvage this limb.

Dr Dholakia, too, was greatly impressed by Govind's courage and the improvement in his infection, and finally said, 'You got a ghost limb to cover with skin, but at least you got away without doing a hindquarter.'

Govind was in hospital for more than two-and-a-half months and all this time, his devoted father camped in his

---

[*] T.E. Udwadia, 'Ghee and Honey Dressing', *Indian Journal of Surgery*, 2011.

car to always be near his son. The day he was discharged, the nurses threw a party. Everyone was happy, but I wondered how useful that right limb, now hanging like the dead branch of a tree, would be to Govind.

But I had not reckoned on Govind's inner strength. He took over his own treatment in Pune. He started daily physiotherapy and weight training and kept at it until he was so exhausted that he couldn't keep awake. He also resumed karate lessons with the sensei that he'd been learning from since he was a child. Govind came to see me every few months. Initially, he used two elbow crutches but after almost a year, to my great joy, he had only one.

At a 1990 conference of the International College of Surgeons—I was then the world president—I postponed my return to Bombay to enable me to attend a lecture on 'Micro vascular nerve transplant' by Professor Hanno Millesi of Vienna the next day. After the lecture, I discussed Govind's case in depth with Prof. Millesi. He was confident that he could replace Govind's sciatic nerve. Both father and son went to Vienna, where Prof. Millesi removed Govind's left sural nerve and used it to bridge the gap in the right sciatic nerve. To ensure that the nerve would be well-covered, vascularized and protected, he also raised a flap of latissimus muscle. Govind had to sleep for several days on his stomach till the nerve graft had taken.

Govind tried out all kinds of treatments, including intensive acupressure therapy. Slowly the nerve graft started taking effect, with Govind initially feeling a tingling sensation in his leg and, ultimately, power in the muscles of his right lower leg. Over the years, he took up several activities to enhance his physical, mental, emotional and spiritual growth, ranging from the meditative technique of Vipassana to scuba diving.

After a few years, he left his family's construction business and branched out on his own. Today, in his late forties, he walks with a barely noticeable limp. He and his daughter run a 65-acre organic farm on the outskirts of Pune where he grows fruits, vegetables and grains. The farm also has a bird sanctuary. He also holds motivational courses and spends a lot of time and money on helping the underprivileged.

Govind gave me the opportunity of witnessing the inspiring journey of a remarkable 18-year-old who went on to live his life to the fullest. I learnt the lesson of a lifetime. From Govind, I learnt that medicine and doctors can only do so much. The patient's real recovery comes from their determination, courage and spiritual strength. I have also learnt to be holistic—whatever helps healing is acceptable and good. Govind has given me faith that god grants miracles to those who deserve them.

11

Surgical Care for the Poor:
A Personal, Indian Perspective

'The future belongs to those who believe in the beauty of their dreams.'

—Eleanor Roosevelt

The current COVID-19 pandemic has changed the world forever. For India, where, in every sphere of life, gross inequalities abound—be it wealth, religion, caste, belief or gender—one clear benefit has emerged: all disparities have been flattened. This catastrophic event has ensured that the rich and the poor, the affluent and the impoverished, all religions and castes have been brought to one level. Many publications have shown that attaining surgical care for the entire population is both affordable and unavoidable because it affects the life of people, their financial status and also defines the national economy. Lack of surgical care accounts for over 2 per cent of the GDP each year. Till last year, health was not a vote bank. Over seventy years and more, each annual budget allocated less than 1 per cent of the GDP for healthcare! Thanks to the pandemic, every government will realize that health may henceforth become the biggest vote bank, for it goes beyond caste, religion, farmers and waivers—it affects every single Indian.

Indian surgery is a two-faced enigma. It lives in a world of make-believe. Surgery done in our cities is equal to, and on occasion better than, that done anywhere else in the world. Our hospital infrastructure and functioning—state-of-the art equipment, often in surplus (India was the largest importer of the robot a few years ago), efficient nurses, surgeons of impeccable quality churning out transplants, minimal access surgery, implants, intraluminal and endoscopic surgery, robotic surgery—offer surgical refinements in every possible speciality. The patient load for surgery in all cities is tremendous and all public hospitals have long waiting lists. Several of our surgeons have international reputations and positions of prestige and power in international surgical bodies. The urban surgeon's heights of achievement, and their continuing thrust for reaching higher, is a matter of great pride and satisfaction. Till 2019, India's medical tourism was increasing at the rate of 15–20 per cent per year. Surgery, as done in the major hospitals of urban India, is the reason why Indian doctors can hold their heads up with pride and say that we are just as good and getting better. This is the face of Indian surgery that the media, healthcare providers, government and medical industry project and promote. *Nothing could be further from the truth.* The other face of Indian surgery is hidden, unseen, unheard and unknown. City surgeons are so involved in their work, progress and recognition that, over the years, they have become unmindful, uncaring and unaware that there is any other surgical world in India except for their own.

I am a city surgeon who worked for over sixty years in tertiary care and teaching hospitals in Mumbai. I have seen that the poor do not only live in rural India. Over 40 per cent of urban people are in a state of deprivation. My ward (Ward 19A) at JJ Hospital had patients on the beds, on mattresses between beds, in corridors and in the main hospital corridor. Lack of infrastructure and an absence of diagnostic facilities accounted for this backlog. Laparoscopy was introduced into Ward 19A and in India for quick diagnosis to improve bed turnover, not as a tribute to technology. Surgeons in cities looked upon diagnostic laparoscopy with scorn. But surgeons in rural India, who had no diagnostic facilities at all, accepted diagnostic laparoscopy and invited me for workshops. The mid-1970s were the peak of India's family-planning programme. Laparoscopes were available in small towns for tubal ligation. This prompted rural surgeons to train for diagnostic laparoscopy.

I am blessed in life. Thanks to laparoscopy, I was granted the opportunity and the privilege to travel extensively around India, in the hope of teaching diagnostic laparoscopy in small-town India. I travelled from east to west, and north to south from 1975 and more so after 1990, with the objective of spreading the gospel of laparoscopic surgery. Believe me, in 1975, Surat was a small town as were Salem and Siliguri. After every visit I made to small-town and rural India to try and teach laparoscopy, I returned humbled, enlightened and educated. I invariably returned from these workshops inspired by the quality, versatility and dedication of rural surgeons. The future of surgery in India as also of the surgical care of the poor lies in the proliferation, education, acknowledgement and recognition of this emerging genre of Indian surgeons who, with courage, capability, innovation, improvisation and sacrifice, have given a new dimension and aura to Indian surgery. In an era where professors in teaching institutions inculcate the importance and cult of sub- and super-specialization to their students in every field, the rural surgeon has shown that, for the vast majority of people and their surgical problems, the ultimate super-specialty is wide-based general surgery. This rural super-specialist will trephine for an extradural, drain an empyema, suture an intestinal perforation, perform a caesarean section, treat a compound fracture and more.

These rural surgeons are prepared to do this because they know that they are the last bastion of the poor, who have travelled long distances to reach them. Beyond them, there is no other succour. Their gains may be meagre but their joys and rewards are bountiful and they may well ask their urban colleagues the question, asked over 2000 years ago, 'What avails a man if he gains the world, but loses his soul?'

My first foray into remote areas was towards the end of 1976, when a group of sixteen surgeons spread out over a 30 km area invited me for a workshop on diagnostic laparoscopy. I am ashamed to admit that I hesitated for a long time to accept their repeated invitations. The workshop was held at the surgeon's residence, which was also his nursing home. There were two generators to provide electricity. As the first day of the workshop was about to get over, a middle-aged patient with acute abdominal pain was admitted. He had travelled for four hours with acute pain that had started two days ago. Clinical examination was strongly in favour of acute appendicitis. There were no investigation facilities. The surgeon felt that he should be operated upon immediately, an opinion with which I agreed. The surgeon gave the spinal anaesthesia, started a drip and gave the anaesthesia monitoring to an unqualified ward boy. Skin preparation was with soap, water and iodine. The instruments and gloves had been sterilized in boiling water over a kerosene Primus stove. The small autoclave could hold only one drum which was packed with two surgeon's gowns and six isolation towels. The gloves must have been used several times before this case. The light was the headlamp of a truck hanging from the ceiling which could be adjusted by a rod from below. The surgeon did a perfect appendectomy with one strand of chromic catgut and cotton thread. Had I not been present, his only assistant would have been an unqualified nurse. The procedure was completed within forty minutes; I could not have done it better. After the workshop the following day, before I returned, I went to see the patient. He was on a soft diet. The patient was indeed blessed that he managed to reach a doctor who was competent after his four-hour pre-operative journey. The doctor came to leave me to the bus stop and, while waiting, I asked him which college he had done his MS from. He told me that he had not done his MS and that he had done his MBBS eighteen years ago. He was keen to progress to laparoscopy. Performance is far more meaningful than a degree.

Atul Gawande in his gripping book *Better*[*] gives a true-to-life account of his two-month tour of hospitals in India, big and small, to see the state of surgical care in India. He writes that the waiting list for surgery at AIIMS, Delhi was around six months, demonstrating the vast load on city hospitals, largely due to a lack of accessible surgical facilities in rural areas. He spent time in the 500-bed public hospital in Nanded where he saw surgeons in the clinics (OPD) and OTs cope smoothly with the variety and pressure of patient load, and dearth of equipment. He wrote with what I feel is admiration tinged with awe, 'How do they do it? How do the surgeons possibly take care of all the hernias, and tumours, the appendicitis cases and kidney stones and manage to sleep, live, survive themselves?' This is why I have, over decades, written that the small-town surgeon is the backbone of Indian surgery.

The solution is in primary care centres—spread out all over the country; mini-hospitals equipped and staffed, from five beds to thirty, depending on the density of the surrounding population. These primary care centres would be more accessible, would look after the hernia, appendicitis and haemorrhoid level of surgeries, thus greatly reducing the horrendous load on hospitals as in Nanded. This is a monumental task to achieve, but only then will the chaos, inequality and inhumanity of surgery for the poor improve.

The steel of the rural Indian surgeon is forged in the strong furnace of deprivation, necessity and want. These have inculcated in them the strength of ingenuity, innovation,

---

[*]   Atul Gawande, *Better* (India: Penguin Books India, 2007).

determination, courage and sacrifice. During every trip when I tried to demonstrate laparoscopy, I was invited to stay in the homes of these warm rural surgeons, each of whom has left a mark on my heart. Today, rural surgery has grown with sophistication because the conditions of rural India have improved so wonderfully—roads, electricity, schools, Internet connection and even Rotary clubs! The entire picture from what it was in 1975 to today has undergone a sea change. Rural surgeons today take pride in what they are doing because they know they are doing surgery which is as good as it is done anywhere, within and beyond the limitations of equipment and facilities. There is far more brotherhood among surgeons in small towns and rural areas. They stick together, help each other and stand by each other. The mental, emotional and professional strength that I have seen in these places is worthy of emulation everywhere. With increasing numbers and self-confidence arising from an awareness of their national importance, these surgeons are gaining in strength, asserting themselves, and have their own association—the Association of Rural Surgeons of India, their own conferences and their own journal. My travels during the call of laparoscopy ensured that I made friends, whom I respected, all over small-town India. One of my highest privileges was to be made an honorary fellow of their association about twenty years ago.

Twenty years back, the editorial board of the *Indian Journal of Surgery*, during my term as chairman/editor, published a special issue on rural surgery in India. Dr R. Tongoankar and his colleagues from different parts of rural India submitted a paper on the repair of hernia using a mosquito net in place of the imported mesh.* The imported mesh cost several hundred rupees and was difficult to get in rural areas, whereas the mosquito net was freely available, and the cost was less than ₹10 per patient, the cost of a cup of tea which any Indian can afford. This group of innovative, enterprising surgeons provided their patients with the gold standard of open hernia repair at a cost affordable to any Indian. I was delighted and proud to publish their paper. Within three weeks, I was castigated by heads of departments of surgery all over India and other teaching institutes for having published an article with no previous scientific data or comparative study and was told that I had degraded the journal by publishing this article. I wrote back asking if scientific data and comparative studies were better suited for a well-financed premier teaching hospital than for a ten-bed nursing home in a rural area. I received no reply. The procedure was ridiculed so much that even rural surgeons fought shy of following it. It is a matter of pride for every Indian surgeon that this mosquito-net repair is today extensively carried out in Africa, South America and Asia.

To try and give this procedure respectability, I had the mosquito net aka mesh studied for all parameters. Having it compared to the imported mesh at the Indian Institute of Technology, Kanpur (IIT-K) which specializes in textiles, I was informed that both the meshes were almost identical in all required studies. I did a comparative study of the two meshes in two Mumbai hospitals and presented the work at

---

* R.R. Tongaonkar, B.V. Reddy and V.K. Mehta, 'Preliminary Multicentre Trial of Cheap Indigenous Mosquito Net Cloth for Tension Free Hernia Repair,' *Indian Journal of Surgery*, 2003.

the International Hernia Conference in Beijing. Most Indian delegates were critical of the use of the mosquito mesh. Dr Pervez Amin, head of the Liechtenstein Institute in Los Angeles where this method had originated, came to my rescue and said that this was an excellent method for poor countries. One of the burdens the rural surgeon carries is that more often than not, their innovations are looked down upon by the pundits of five-star hospitals.

I must emphasize that during my visit to small-town and rural India, I saw what surgery was available because I only visited places for a workshop where surgeons were present over an area of 30–50 km in fair number. I have not seen the true vast interior, where no surgeon is present over a 100 km area—the horrors and miseries of grassroots rural India. The Lancet Commission on Rural Surgeries, 2015, informs that in Moderate-to-Low Income Countries (MLIC) of which India is one, *5 billion people lack access to safe, affordable surgical care* when needed. A patient with a strangulated hernia or a lady with obstructed labour could die without seeing a doctor, leave alone a surgeon. That is the destitute, deprived and desolate India we need to address.

Over the last three years, the government has announced a very commendable, timely and ambitious scheme—the Ayushman Bharat scheme for *universal health coverage*, to meet *sustainable development goals* (SDGs) and the *commitment to leave no one behind*, three worthy objectives. It has two components—health wellness centres and the Pradhan Mantri Jan Arogya Yojana. To the credit of this government, this is the first national health scheme this country has seen over seventy years and came into action much before the pandemic. The healthcare centres aim to 'transform' 1.5 lakh primary health centres to keep people healthy and choose healthy behaviour. The terms 'healthy' and 'choose healthy behaviour' are vague and carry little meaning or impact. This could well end up in 1.5 lakh concrete structures without any planning, devoid of infrastructure or adequate equipment, where the doctor is absent 46 per cent of the time and, when present, is frequently incapable to deal with the situation. *A primary care centre needs professional planning, meticulous execution, infrastructure and equipment, and manpower allocations. Most of all, it needs not empty promises, but honest, total government commitment.*

If the government means business to leave no one behind, it should ensure that every health welfare centre or primary healthcare centre, whatever you call it, should:

1. be within timely reach of the population,
2. be well-planned to function as a mini-hospital and have complete infrastructure in terms of equipment and facilities,
3. be staffed by trained and committed personnel for safe and effective cure, and
4. ensure that the treatment will be affordable to a poor family.

This will obviously entail a tremendous cost, but surgical interventions are cost-effective and investments for surgery at the primary level have been found and proven to be affordable. Limited and Minimal Income Countries like Mongolia, Mexico and more than fifteen other MLICs are rapidly moving towards attaining this goal. Why should India be left behind? If the government is straining every sinew over infrastructure for toilets, water, banking, Internet and digitalization for all, why not create infrastructure for health and surgery for all?

Anyone involved in surgical care in India should study the Lancet Commission on Global Surgery released in 2015. Not only is there a strong argument in favour of strengthening surgical infrastructure, but it is demonstrated that doing so will improve both the health of the people and the economy. If, at the primary health centre, what is termed as bellwether conditions can be satisfactorily and safely carried out, it would ensure that *80 per cent of surgical care in India could be met at the peripheral level.* The three requirements of the bellwether are: the surgeons should be capable of doing a caesarean section, of looking after a compound fracture and treating an acute abdomen. If infrastructure is made available in terms of manpower and equipment for just these three conditions, it would cover almost 80 per cent of all surgeries because these three conditions represent the requirements of the greater part of surgical care. Lancet Global Health 2015 reports that 30 per cent of the global burden of disease is due to surgically treatable conditions.[*] One can appreciate the burden of surgical care that goes unrecognized and untreated in this country. Bringing universal surgical care to India is a humongous problem and a massive undertaking. If we have the combined will to do it, if we have the capacity to reach for the moon and Mars, if we have the capacity to give the Internet to our villages, I am sure we have the capacity to fulfil this important humanitarian responsibility. This can only be done as a *national enterprise,* akin to the infrastructure projects for roads and railways. It requires all hands on deck—with the government leading the initiative and coordinating with public and private sector agencies, public health associations, surgical

---

[*]   M.G. Shrime, S.W. Bickler, B.C. Alkire and C. Mock, 'Global Burden of Surgical Disease', *Lancet Global Health*, 2015.

associations, medical associations, anaesthesia associations as well as both rural and urban surgeons—for this project to be a success. What we require is that there should be safe and affordable aid and support within timely reach of the population. The accessibility to the centre is essential. A study has shown that patients with acute abdomen, who are 100 km from a hospital that can give safe treatment, have sixteen times greater mortality then those within reasonable reach, which shows the importance of accessibility.

The first step is to recognize the fact that there is an unmet, large burden of surgical patients who receive no surgical aid and that this is the highest form of inequality in healthcare. The mortality from this unmet surgical care in India is greater than the mortality of HIV, tuberculosis and malaria put together. The next step is for a strong governmental health body dedicated to this cause, which would act like a corporate body to administrate this scheme, to ensure adequate funds, an efficient supply chain of equipment and material, and efficient distribution of the workforce, which would be kept motivated by adequate financial returns, incentives, promotions and appreciation. Discipline must be ensured in every cadre of the staff; there must be financial transparency and maintenance of statistics to ensure the efficient and cost-effective running of this gigantic project.

The second part of the Ayushman Bharat scheme is what is described as the world's largest insurance system for surgical care, giving surgical cover to crores of the marginalized poor. This is very commendable and a tremendous support to crores of the poor, but remains a substantial annual expenditure that will recur every year. Further, transferring this surgical load to urban hospitals adds to the already heavy burden of routine surgery in our cities. One of the aims of Ayushman Bharat is the achievement of Sustainable Development Goals. There is a saying that if you give a fish to a person, you feed them for one day, but if you teach the person to fish and give them the implements to fish, they will eat for the rest of their lives. We need sustainable permanent development.

When the government proposed to permit surgical postgraduates from the AYUSH system (traditional Indian medical schools: Ayurveda, Yoga and Naturopathy, Unani, Siddha and Homeopathy) with equivalent surgical privileges as the allopathic system, the Indian Medical Association (IMA), Medical Council of India (MCI) and every surgical association went up in arms that this would jeopardize patient safety. I agree that it certainly would. But let us get off our high horse that allopaths are an intellectually superior race. Why did several of these individuals become AYUSH surgeons? Not by choice but by necessity, possessing the motivation and determination to become doctors and surgeons but not getting admission to MBBS courses, which forced them into the AYUSH system. My teacher, Dr A.V. Baliga, could not get admission for an MBBS because his Udupi matriculation was not accepted by the British. He became an AYUSH doctor. He scrounged for loans, went to London, did his London matriculation, then the LRCP, MRCS and, finally, FRCS, to fulfil his dream of becoming a surgeon and he was one of the best in the country. I have had, for long, several resident surgeons in Mumbai hospitals from AYUSH. They work with as much ability and commitment, assist at surgery equally well, and are reliable and efficient. Over 60 per cent of rural patients in India are treated by totally unqualified health practitioners, some *vaid*s, some quacks, who presumably are a greater threat than AYUSH.

Surely we should be just as worried about them as we are about the AYUSH doctors. We conveniently turn a blind eye to them. Let us be realistic. With full government recognition, we cannot merely wish AYUSH away. We need to keep our perspective and priorities right. *Every surgeon in India counts* (I sometimes ask myself whether we should train suitable MBBS doctors in surgery, but I do not want to stir another hornet's nest right now). I am sure even the AYUSH surgeons know their limitations. In the national interest, we must help try to bridge the gap so that AYUSH surgeons can perform safe, basic surgery, treat a compound fracture, do a caesarean or a laparotomy, and tend to peripheral centres which are going a-begging for surgeons. *Can this be achieved?* There are pitfalls and hurdles in bridging with AYUSH, problems ranging from training in safety, looking after one's turf, to ego. Getting AYUSH to fit the bill is a major problem but let us, as surgeons, accept that every problem we face in our day-to-day surgery must have a solution. It is mandatory that rural surgeons are given the same respect and acknowledgement as urban surgeons, with fitting, appropriate financial status to ensure that they are happy and content in their work and minimize attrition.

In summary, we need to make sure that we have a permanent solution to surgical healthcare and that permanent solution is to take healthcare where it is needed and where there is none—in rural India. Surgical care for the poor is an uphill and herculean task and yet, a task worthy of every ounce of our collective effort and energy. It is vital that every government source, be it the Centre or the state, the private sector, every association and all doctors, from professors to village doctors, pool their concerns in this effort. A sincere effort and success in this cause would, by far, be the greatest triumph and the ultimate success story in the history of surgery so as to ensure surgical care for all. This utopian dream may take years or even decades, but when the fundamental right to surgical healthcare and to all healthcare is met, India will be a fair, just and better country.

'Our doubts are traitors and make us lose the good we oft might win, by fearing to attempt.'

—W. Shakespeare

12

The Making of a Surgeon

Disclaimers always come at the end but are seldom noticed, which is why I decided to start with one to make sure it is read. The author wishes to make it abundantly clear that this chapter is merely a collection of his own thoughts, experiences, fears and failures that span nearly seventy years of surgery. While on no account does he claim any special expertise on this subject, approximately seven decades of surgical experience have given him the opportunity to learn things that can't be found in textbooks or taught in medical schools. It is with humility that he wishes to present these thoughts.

The image that many patients and, dare I say, some surgeons have of a surgeon is one of a prima donna with virtuoso hands, who single-handedly swoops in and magically extricates life from the jaws of death. They are seen as performing miracles—and performing them alone—with the odds usually stacked against them. When it comes to great surgeons, the focus is invariably on operating, but after almost seventy years in the profession, I can tell you that this is simply not true. When I appeared for my pilot's exam in 1962, flying a Piper Cub, I thought I flew the best flight of my life. I jumped out from the cockpit and extended my hand to accept the examiner's congratulations. He took my hand reluctantly saying that I had, in fact, failed my test because I read out the checklist as though it was an unnecessary formality. Just as he told me that there was more to being a pilot than flying a plane, I also learnt over time that there was more to being a surgeon than simply performing operations.

After studying my own surgery, seeing my peers and seeing the quality of excellent surgeons in India and overseas, I have come to the conclusion that there are only five essential requirements to make a good surgeon:

1. Honesty
2. Humility
3. Empathy
4. Passion
5. Leadership

I feel that all the other attributes can be loaded on this foundation of honesty, humility, empathy, passion and leadership.

Over the last several decades, many residents have come to me at the end of their term, asking me for specific advice that I can give them for becoming a good surgeon. I usually give them one piece of advice, which is to *just be yourself.* If you are authentically yourself and do things with integrity, you will never do any wrong to any patient in any way. Accept current teachings if *you* feel they are right and in the patient's interest and keep on hold what you cannot decide. You could possibly be wrong in what you accept or reject—that is inevitable—but at least it is a decision you made with the best interests of your patients at heart. This is easier said than done: being yourself is not as comfortable as going along with the herd, but I promise you that it will give you inner peace all throughout your life. It will also be the only way you will grow. I have been ridiculed, humiliated and abused because laparoscopy, at the time when I was using it extensively, was not the established way of doing things. India is now a world leader in laparoscopic procedures.

Dr Eric Muhe, who did the first laparoscopic cholecystectomy in 1985, was a small-town surgeon in Germany who just wanted to be himself and follow a path he believed in. His professors, intolerant of his heterodox surgery, rewarded him for his efforts by having him tried for manslaughter, where he was subjected to a process that included trial, bail and jail that went on for five years. Until his reputation was resurrected by international surgeons and he was given his deserved place in history, he continued to remain true to himself even in oblivion. I had the opportunity to become his friend in 2000, just before I gave the Millennium SAGES lecture at the SAGES annual conference.* Dr Muhe had given the same lecture the previous year, which I had not heard. I wrote to him for a copy of his lecture, 'Roadblocks to Surgical Progress'. He wrote back at length about his experiences. The humility and strength

---

* T.E. Udwadia, 'Millennium Lecture. One World—One People—One Surgery,' *Surgical Endoscopy*, 2001.

of a man who had fashioned the instrument for the world's first laparoscopic cholecystectomy from his daughter's bicycle tubing came through in his letters.

This also brings me to something that has perplexed me often enough to mention it in these pages. Every surgeon, without exception, should be humble because we are repeatedly given reasons to be so. No surgeon is free of making mistakes and every mistake is a call for humility. Strangely, humility is hard for some surgeons to accept and the near holy reverence given to them, coupled with their own personal assessment of their superhuman prowess, endorses hubris and suppresses humility.

If any surgeon says they don't make mistakes, they have not done enough surgery or are losing their memory. And every mistake is an opportunity. If they accept their blunder and realize what caused it, and put the entire episode into memory for future reference, it will not be repeated. In a sticky surgical situation, recalling your past missteps is key to the success of the procedure. In Ward 19A of JJ Hospital, my senior colleague Dr Rasik Patel would tell every new batch of residents who came to our unit that there are three types of surgeons:

1. Those who learn by other surgeons' mistakes
2. Those who learn by their own mistakes
3. Those who just don't

Humility ensures that the surgeon knows their limits and is willing to accept, learn and move on. While the arrogant may conflate this quality with weakness, it takes a special kind of strength to know yourself, know your worth and judge your capacity.

Dr George Berci is considered by most as one of the leading surgeons of our time and is widely attributed as a visionary, innovator and inventor in the fields of endoscopy and laparoscopy since 1962. Laparoscopy is one of the only three true patient-friendly advances ever made in surgery (the other two are anaesthesia and asepsis, which has removed the morbidity and mortality of post-operative infection). To me, he is an icon of humility. I first met Dr Berci in 1990 at the SAGES conference in Atlanta. He was not what I thought he would be—he was not much over 5 feet tall and was frail with bushy, enquiring eyebrows. I gave him a hug and realized that genius comes in all shapes and sizes.

Over the years, I learnt his life story. George was born in Hungary before the Second World War. Being Jewish, at the age of 23, he was forcibly packed into a train with other Jews headed to a concentration camp from which very few came out alive. Along the way, near Budapest, there was heavy aerial bombing which forced the train to stop and the guards to run for shelter. He escaped and reached Budapest where he worked for the Hungarian underground, forging passports for escaping Jews. While his dream was to become a musician, at the end of the war, he became a doctor as that was his mother's wish. And what a glittering career he had! Within three years of graduating medical school, he set up the first experimental surgery department in Budapest. Later, over a ten-year period in Melbourne, he drew global attention to his work on the engineering aspects, instrumentation and concepts of endoscopy. The American College of Surgeons (ACS) awarded him with their highest honour, the Jacobson Innovation Award, while SAGES established the George Berci Lifetime Achievement Award.

In all the time that I knew him, he never mentioned his vast contributions to surgery. When we got together he usually discussed the future, his appreciation of his colleagues, his joy in playing the violin or the exploits of his beloved wife Barbara. In 2013, I received the George Berci Lifetime Achievement Award from SAGES, which I consider to be a singular honour. Many surgeons, such as George, are not even aware of their humility for it comes so naturally to them, giving them the freedom to constantly improve themselves, which will ensure exponential surgical growth and leadership.

I also found Dr Berci to be empathetic which, in my view, is a quality that is vital for a surgeon. I still remember my time as a registrar at KEM when we lost three open-heart surgery patients to different post-operative complications in one night. At that time, there was no ICU where the patient could be hidden from the family. All three patients were in the general ward within a few beds of one another, with members of the family in attendance. The families were witness to the frantic external cardiac massages, the intubation and the maniacal attempts to keep the patients alive with an Ambu bag (there was no ventilator then). They could also see the two-minute instant venesection we performed for a collapsed patient with no pulse, no veins, pushing adrenaline directly into the heart, all in a dimly-lit, over-congested ward. And, eventually, the futility of it all.

While Sharad was doing the paperwork, I had to meet the families. Empathy has particular importance when the surgeon has the task of giving bad news to the family. Relatives can tell the difference between a set and practised apology and true empathy, which softens the blow. Each family, almost within an hour of each other, lost a member. One of the senior family members bent to touch my feet, which I stopped immediately. He then held my hand and expressed the family's gratitude for our efforts. I learnt that language and words do not convey empathy; it is true sorrow, the expression, the eyes and the body language that give solace to the family. Every family—rich or poor, educated or illiterate—can tell the difference between true empathy and a well-rehearsed act.

To my mind, everyone can cultivate empathy but you can't cultivate anything if you don't have strong passion. Passion is what gives flight to the surgeon's curiosity in looking for new advances; it is the fire in the surgeon's belly, the fuel in their tank, giving them the thrust to increase their reach. As I witnessed working in Prof. Sen's department, passion can compensate for limited resources. It is the future of surgery because it pushes the envelope. It doesn't matter if you're a surgeon or an IT professional or someone who bakes cakes for a living. What most professions have in common is that they are evolving all the time, and it is up to you to be up to date with your skills. It's also important for surgeons to critique and audit their own work at regular intervals. For example, the gold standard of hernia procedures was set decades ago. It's possible for a surgeon doing the same procedure over and over again to become complacent, and perhaps even regress. The surgeon must not fall into this trap.

To illustrate just what passion can do, in the annals of the history of surgery there is no better example than the story of organ transplantation. Surgeons from many parts of the world dedicated a large part of their lives over decades— sometimes at their personal and financial cost—towards making organ transplantation a reality, saving millions of lives. Thomas Starzl was one such pioneer who developed a technique in dogs which, even today, is the method for liver transplant in humans.

But it was not an easy road. While Starzl was internationally recognized for his work, there was no success in liver transplantation. He had the courage to stop his work on the liver for over three years because he realized that the only way to the liver was through the kidney. The beauty is that all surgeons who were passionate about transplant surgery had the honesty and goodwill to keep exchanging notes with each other, trying to improve each other's knowledge and experience through combined efforts. This was an important factor in making organ transplantation possible. Starzl led the pack. Roy Calne from Cambridge informed Starzl that, in dog experiments, donor kidney survival was improved with the use of the immune suppressant cyclosporine. Starzl confirmed this, but reasoned that cyclosporine needed something more to ensure better kidney survival. He added steroids, saw the improvement and took this into clinical practice. At one time, he had the largest number of living kidney transplant survivors in the world. With success in the kidney transplant, Starzl returned to his liver programme with renewed passion. The head of surgery at a Denver hospital for nearly two decades, he left in 1980 under stressful and traumatic conditions, unsure of where he would go next. He started working in Pittsburgh with no designation and no department, taking only two members from his Denver team with him. It was in Pittsburgh that Starzl reaped the rewards of unending frustration, bitterness and stress; months, years and decades spent in the dog lab; and the psychological trauma of patients lost on the way, which hit him very hard. Liver transplantations zoomed like a rocket. It was primarily through his determination and passion that liver transplants became part of practical surgery.

Manual dexterity is vital to a surgeon's performance during surgery. If all unfavourable outcomes are analysed, roughly 30 per cent are due to manual error, and the remaining 70 per cent are caused by mistakes not attributable to the surgeon's hand. These are the errors of skills not taught at training centres or by didactic lectures but instead are picked up during residencies to include cognitive and interpersonal errors like decision making, adaptability and stress management, among others.

At the start of my first house post, my registrar told me that he would not let me hold the scalpel till I could tie fast, fluent and safe knots. I took thread from the OT and practised tying knots for hours on the back of the chair in my room till I literally couldn't see my fingers move and the back of the chair looked like a white wig. I got a chance to hold the scalpel but the next requirement was to tie knots around an artery forceps deep in the corner of the pocket of my hospital apron. This sounds so primitive in comparison to today's advanced training in manual dexterity, but it served the purpose over sixty years ago. And the best thing about manual dexterity is that it can be achieved even if the surgeon doesn't have a natural gift for it. As the chairman of the Centre of Excellence for Minimal Access Surgery Training (ceMAST), one of the world's most outstanding training centres, I saw over 8000 surgeons trained in a dozen surgical specialities on dry models, animal models and through virtual reality. I have seen beginners struggling to develop hand-eye coordination and yet, with diligent practice and expert mentoring, acquire manual dexterity. With practice and patience and, of course, correct instructions, anything is possible.

The surgeon must be a pathological perfectionist with attention to the minutest details. I teach all students that there are only four essential requirements for taking a good stitch in any part of the body:

1. Equal distance on both sides of the cut
2. Equal depth on both sides of the cut
3. Right angles to the cut surface
4. Bringing the cut surfaces together gently by approximation and not by strangulation

While I don't suture skin as often as I used to, I try to make it a teaching example when I do. I intentionally place a poor stitch, go to the next stitch, complete it and then come back and remove the improper stitch to impress on the residents that there is no shame in undoing something that has not been properly done. The message goes home: it is not a matter of shame but a credit to undo unacceptable work. Precision is all-important. Today, most intestinal anastomoses are done with staplers, but I feel that a hand-sewn anastomosis is more gratifying and an excellent exercise in precision. The precision should be such that it would appear that the suturing has been done by a Singer sewing machine. For that matter, when I am doing an intestinal anastomosis, I mutter under my breath, 'Good, good, good, reasonable, perfect, perfect, shitty stitch!' and I compensate for that shitty stitch with a neat one. Every surgeon has their own method of attaining concentration and perfection and this is mine.

Shitty stitch or not, the buck stops with the surgeon, and having a sense of accountability is crucial. There is nothing more pathetic and pitiable than a surgeon who shouts, throws tantrums and instruments, blames the nurse, lights, the assistant or anything else that moves or doesn't move in the OT. Every team needs to have a captain and, in surgery, the leader is obviously the surgeon. All surgeons are not cut out to be leaders, but it is surprising how so many of them grow into the role. The surgeon may call for an opinion but the final call is theirs and that is where they prove their worth with judgement and wisdom. The leader not only leads with mastery in surgery but with their character, ethical code and approach to everyone in their environment. They should talk as softly and gently with the theatre assistant as they would with a senior colleague. Leadership is a heavy mantle and requires broad shoulders.

Having said that, leadership and teamwork go hand-in-hand. The surgeon must have respect for the entire team, know each team member's strengths and weaknesses and learn how to accept both differing views and justified criticism. Communication must be clear, firm, soft, easy to understand and to the point.

But the proof of true leadership is, of course, in a crisis. A sudden disaster in the OT may give you a sense of panic but it's best to keep your voice soft, your movements measured and your brain sharp and alert. Your heart will be racing, trying to press the recall button in your brain to mine the data stored from past experiences, and retrieve the required solution for this particular situation. A suggestion given should be carefully and swiftly considered and the decision has to be almost instantaneous. It cannot be made later, not tomorrow, not after going to the library or consulting friends. That's why it's so important to learn from your past mistakes and tap into those experiences when you need them. Recall saves lives.

The patient and the surgeon have a combined journey of which the operation is an important vital event, but they travel together before and after the surgery. Over the last twenty-odd years, I find that the first consultations are becoming more difficult. As one gets older, the surgeon finds that they are not the first port-of-call. The patient has seen other surgeons before and all investigations and files—and sometimes even Google printouts—are brought and placed on the table, and they look expectantly at the surgeon, presuming all that material will be studied. After smiling and asking the patient and accompanying people to sit (I formerly used to stand up if a lady was present; now, I merely make a pretence of standing because of my knee and back pain), I gently push back the pile of paperwork, saying that these are pieces of paper and images of X-rays. *I am not treating your reports, I am treating you*, is what I tell them. *Tell me about your case from the beginning.*

Earlier, patients were happy to talk and often had to be curbed. Today's patients are hesitant about this 'new' way of examination. As the patient starts talking, I start writing, interspersing our time together with questions. When the history of the illness is complete, I have written about twenty lines, and it has taken a few minutes. As we talk, the ice is broken and we get friendlier. By the time we go through the personal history of diet, alcohol, smoking and exercise, history of illness and come to family history, the patient and companions are eager to talk. My first page—the history—is complete. In the process, we have spoken about children, education, sports, what food they like and so on, and a gentle bond is created. After their BP is taken, I hold the patient's wrist for some time. I may not be taking the pulse, just talking. My father had taught me that mere skin contact with the patient creates a bond. And the wrist is the most innocuous place to hold the patient.

This first consultation is an essential step in the making of a surgeon. Investigations must be minimal and pertinent to the case. A flurry of investigations, many of them unrequired, do not impress the intelligent patient, and add significantly to their financial burden. The first consultation is the cornerstone of the patient–surgeon partnership and both the patient and their family must leave with confidence and trust in the surgeon. At the next consultation, if surgery is required, the description of the surgery must be given honestly, complete with possible adverse effects so that the patient knows what to expect. Truth creates trust. It is wrong to say that this or that is a small procedure and that the patient should not worry. There is no 'minor surgery' in my vocabulary.

The relationship and the bond should continue with post-operative care. A sense of humour goes a long way. While this may sound vain, I find that in my own experience—after having been through eight operations myself—the most important event the patient looks forward to, for the next twenty-four hours, is the surgeon's visit. Patients should be reassured, listened to and, most importantly, cheered up. I make it a point to find out about the important investigations before I enter so that I don't have to look at the sheet again in front of the patient. The patient wants you to talk to them, to listen to them and not just look at the reports. They want to tell you how their twenty-four hours have been and it is your duty to listen. However late you may be, never give your patient the impression that you are in a hurry. I have a standing instruction for every resident in every hospital over decades—if they leave the patient's room without making the patient smile or laugh, or feel better after their visit, about their visit, they might as well have not come. Up until about ten years ago, I would visit every patient I had operated on that day, after my consultation, before going home. I felt that the patient slept better after having seen me. I know that I slept far better for having seen the patient.

Of course, the ultimate proof of all surgical efforts is only one: the outcome. The outcome is what defines the quality of the surgeon, their team and the hospital, but operative skills are not the only component. Other important contributors can be divided into cognitive/mental and interpersonal/social. The skills include knowledge, decision-making, planning, situational awareness, adaptation, anticipation, stress management, ingenuity and being positive, among several other attributes. All of these, in tandem, help surgeons take the right calls. A good result should be topmost on the mind at the first consultation, through the investigation, the surgery and the follow-up period. Because the outcome is what matters most to the patient.

So, ultimately, what makes a surgeon? Just as all patients are not the same, all surgeons are not the same. Before anaesthesia is started on my patient, I invariably remove my mask, much to the annoyance of every OT nurse. The patient, even if sedated, is lying on a table, petrified, with four or five masked people standing around looking at them—no less than a scene from a horror movie. To see my face, the only face they know, and hopefully like and trust (the importance of the first consultation), is comforting. If, as a bonus, the surgeon is holding the patient's hand, saying, 'Think happy thoughts and go to sleep' when going under, all is well. Each time I have needed an operation, I have chosen my own surgeon with care. Having worked with most of them, I know their qualities of hand, head and heart. So far, I have been right in my selection. A good surgeon is god's gift to the patient.

While we're on the subject of god, I do feel that religion has a great part to play in surgery. And by religion, I mean faith. I am not overtly religious, and ten minutes of prayer after my bath is sufficient for me. But when I am scrubbing for surgery, the whole team knows that I am to be left to myself. While scrubbing, I recite the simplest of all Zoroastrian prayers, and often a request to St Jude. This short prayer— scrubbing is getting shorter with new anti-microbial agents—is for the welfare of the patient I am operating on. I get strength, confidence and results because of this short expression of faith. We surgeons sometimes are so full of our own image, that we forget that all good things come from above. In my study at home, I have had, for over forty years, a plaque that sets up my day: *Lord, help me to remember that nothing is going to happen to me today that You and I together can't handle.* No matter how committed and experienced I may hope to be, I have never taken credit for saving a patient's life because I truly believe that lives are not saved by us; lives are saved by a higher power.

13

A Surgeon's Journey

'Travellers, there is no path; paths are made by walking.'

—Antonio Machado

My surgical journey began as an undergraduate student at GS Medical College—students on surgical rotation were termed 'surgical dressers', which made us feel superior to students doing a medical rotation who were called 'medical clerks'. In the second week of my first surgical rotation, the house surgeon told me to stay with the patient who was receiving a blood transfusion that he had started in the side OT of the Jan Mohamed Theatre, while he completed his ward work.

In those days, doctors were required to stay with the patient till the transfusion was over. Today, when I think of my first assignment, I feel that it was such an overkill for a procedure carried out routinely now by nurses and ward assistants. But in 1953, a blood transfusion was more than a procedure, it was an event. For me, this incident remains the best example of the advances made in surgery over the last seventy-odd years, more than what have been seen in the millennia before.

When I would visit my father's dispensary in the 1950s, glass syringes and steel needles were sterilized in boiling water for reuse—a practice followed by all major hospitals of that time—but this method would unwittingly be the cause of the spread of hepatitis B and C. Even during my first-ever surgical experience of the blood transfusion mentioned above, the blood would slowly drip, drop by drop, through a red rubber tube which would again be sterilized by boiling. While that particular patient didn't have a reaction, many others did—caused more due to the rubber tube than the transfusion itself.

I still remember my first viewing of a major surgery—as an undergraduate student, getting a bird's-eye view from the viewing gallery of the Jan Mohamed Theatre where Dr Munsif was doing a splenectomy. As the incision was deepened, every single bleeding vessel was caught in a haemostat (artery forceps) to stop the bleeding and the haemostats were left in place, so that by the time the abdomen was opened, there were well over a few dozen haemostats hanging from both sides of the incision. This made a very dramatic sight. I was very impressed. After the spleen was removed, the haemostats were removed one by one, starting from the deeper part of the incision till the skin. The haemostats had been in position for over two hours. When they were removed, most of the blood vessels had been sealed. The few that were still bleeding after removing the haemostats were ligated with cotton thread. Time was not wasted in tying every haemostat. Historically, this method of haemostasis would now be equivalent to a silent black-and-white movie in cinema. While electrocautery was available at that time, it was so erratic that it was used to the minimum. This could be because unpredictable cautery could suddenly burn a large area of tissue. In addition, the rubber gloves were reused several times and had small punctures, which gave painful electric shocks to the surgical team.

Today's surgeons often talk about robotics and organ transplants, or cite the intersection of technology and surgery as proof of how far we have come. They may well laugh at me for placing the introduction of plastics in surgery—disposable syringes, IV lines and other uses—or new energy sources on an equal footing, but it is both my view and my experience that these relatively humble advances affect far more lives than more state-of-the-art developments.

Sterile plastic tubing as well as sterile disposable syringes and needles have all been advances benefiting the safety, welfare and lives of billions of people and have also been revolutionary in terms of the changes they've introduced to the quality of patient care and outcomes. In comparison, the robot or the stapler have helped but only a minuscule part of the population, and have made notable but not total changes to patient outcome. Technology that benefits a limited number of patients catches the public eye, but the quiet advance which benefits every single human is not to be scoffed at. Ask those who have struggled through rubber tubes, boiled syringes, blunt needles and non-functional cautery.

While extolling the growth made over the last seventy years, one cannot give enough credit to two seminal advances made from 1840 to 1860—anaesthesia and asepsis. Anaesthesia converted surgery from a savage assault to a somewhat humane science and asepsis ensured that the patient would be protected from mortality and high morbidity due to sepsis. It was only after the combination of these two advances that it was possible to even attempt surgery in the abdomen, chest or head.

It also may be meaningful to note that every advance has had the welfare of the patient as its sole objective. If it helped the surgeon or the doctor, it was fortuitous and not the original intention. Specifically, all the progress made in surgery has been multidirectional, holistic and forward-looking in every aspect of patient care, starting with the prevention of surgery in the first place. Prophylactic care, for example—like the campaign against tobacco or regular screening for disease detection— helps keep surgical intervention at bay.

But not all advances were initially welcome. There was strong opposition to specialization to start with. General surgeons would feel they could do a gastrectomy or a nephrectomy just as well as a specialist, and wanted to protect their turf. But over time, the specialists proved themselves with better outcomes. The case for specialization was further underscored during my experience with Aditya, a fourteen-year-old boy born with a duodenal atresia (a congenital closure of the small intestine just beyond the stomach, preventing the stomach contents from moving forward).

He had his first surgery when he was just a day old and this was followed up by subsequent surgeries. When I first saw him, he had not retained solids over a period of time, not even water by mouth. A tall, strapping boy of over 6 feet, his weight had swiftly dropped from 72 kg to 40 kg—he was a sleeping skeleton. His father expected me to operate immediately and became highly agitated when I told him I would only do so when the patient was fit for surgery. Total Parenteral Nutrition (TPN) was started through a neck IV and Dr Mangal Jain worked with him to bring him up to the appropriate metabolic, electrolyte and nutritional balance. Chest physiotherapy and exercise was started. Each day on rounds, I would sit and chat with him to de-stress him, sometimes smuggling in some chocolate to bring a smile to his face.

Though I ran the self-created tertiary care GI and HPB (Hepato-Pancreato-Biliary) surgery unit at JJ Hospital and was a founder member of HPB International, I was still a general surgeon and was certain Aditya's re-surgery would be difficult. To that end, I requested a trained GI specialist, Dr Nilesh Doctor, to help me, and he graciously accepted my request. The surgery was tricky from the start. Loops of bowel were densely stuck to each other all over the abdomen. Trying to separate the adhesions would start serosal tears in the bowel wall. While it was eventually completed with difficult bowel reconstruction, I was glad that I requested a specialist like Nilesh to scrub in. There is no place for ego in surgery.

In the mid-1970s to the early 1980s, only a handful of surgeons scattered across India were taking special interest in GI and HPB surgery but they were working in isolation: B.M.L. Kapoor and Samiran Nandy from Delhi, N. Rangabashyam and B. Krishna Rao from Chennai, Amrish Parikh from Ahmedabad, V.N. Shrikande and myself from Mumbai and, similarly, a few from Vellore, Chandigarh and Lucknow. The only way we could exchange information at that time was to visit each other at our hospitals and see each other's work.

It was left to N. Rangabashyam to take the bold step—in the face of significant opposition to specialization—and set up the first department of GI and HPB surgery at Madras Medical College to establish GI surgery in India. From this early nucleus has grown the large active body of Indian GI HPB surgery.

In Aditya's post-operative course, the gastric aspiration remained at over 2000 ml daily for seven days. There was no peristaltic activity in the abdomen. I was worried that the operative procedure had not served its purpose. On the tenth day, the patient's father insisted on another surgery and it was hard to pacify him. On the fourteenth day, the aspiration abruptly dropped to 400 ml and he passed some gas. The improvement was progressive and the operation was eventually a success. Four to five years later, Aditya went on to top engineering college, makes time for football, and is a strapping boy at 6'2" and 78 kg. To my mind, this case also underscores the advance of surgery. Aditya was not saved by the surgeon or the operation but by the progressive advance of surgery in a multidimensional manner. He was optimally prepared for surgery with excellent medical management and brought to the ideal physiological balance. Skilful anaesthesia by Dr Vazifdar and Dr Bhagat exemplified a significant advance in all supporting specialities. His tailor-made post-operative management was also a life-giving surgical advance. Today, with the exception of extreme emergencies, every patient is prepped for surgery by bringing them to an optimal level for respiratory-pulmonary function, nutrition, metabolic balance and whatever else may be required.

Another advance that was initially unwelcome was laparoscopy or minimal access surgery (MAS). Starting in 1972, it was an integral part of my journey. Unacceptable at first by the professors and the teaching establishment who were prisoners of evidence-based medicine, it was the benefit of laparoscopy to patient recovery and early return to activity that led *patients* to push for this technique. Surgical training to cope with the demands of MAS became the need of the hour and this resulted in a great change in surgical thinking and performance. Instrumentation and new procedures do not make the patient safe. It's the surgeon who makes the instrumentation and new procedures safe.

The motto of my alma mater G.S. Medical College is something I have always lived by: 'You are here not to worship what is taught but to question it.' Questioning things rather than blindly accepting them has been an integral part of my journey, be it for advancing the cause of laparoscopy or using ghee and honey dressings or promoting the use of mosquito net meshes for hernia repair. The criticism I initially faced was eventually all for a good cause because in surgery, truth often starts off as blasphemy.

Both teaching and learning have always been a passion for me, from the time I was a registrar at KEM and Royal Liverpool. At that time, there was no Internet—surgical journals were the chief sources of information and these were usually two years out of date. To close this gap, from 1973, I decided to take a sabbatical every year for my own education and bring back my learnings to India. I visited Harold Ellis—now Sir Harold—at Westminster Hospital, London. Mr Ellis was—and is—considered to be one of England's best surgery teachers. At ninety-three, he still teaches anatomy at Oxford. A ward round with him was an unforgettable lesson in bedside teaching.

I also had a sabbatical with John Goligher at Leeds Infirmary to see all sequential variants of vagotomy which he performed along with sphincter-saving colon surgery. With no video transmission, the only way to see these legends operate was to be in the OT, in your street clothes and shoes, standing on wooden platforms to get a glimpse. When I visited Prof. Goligher, there was a large blackboard in the OT with the figure 189 written in bold letters. The next day, the figure was 188, and then 187 the following day. Intrigued, I asked about the blackboard. Goligher said the nurses were reminding him of the number of days left for him to retire. Perhaps it was because he would operate from eight to eight!

I visited Irvine Lichtenstein twice in Los Angeles—for the first time in 1978, to see how he did his anatomic inguinal hernia repair under local anaesthesia. The second time was in 1984, which was the year he first started the tension-free mesh repair, the gold standard for open hernia surgery today. I learnt it and brought back the exact technique to teach my residents.

A stint in Kiel with the legendary laparoscopic gynaecologist Dr Kurt Semm helped cement my fundamentals in laparoscopy. A pioneering surgeon, he was also the inventor of laparoscopic equipment like the insufflator. Before the advent of camera surgery, he improvised and had a stand fitted to the operation table which held the telescope, so that both his hands were free to operate. He had a teaching attachment fitted to the eyepiece through which I could see him operate—stupid moron that I was, I did not bring this concept to India.

In addition to a wonderful sabbatical with Dr Starzl in Denver in the US for liver transplants, I also had the privilege to spend some time with Prof. Thompson at St Mark's Hospital, London, the mecca for colorectal surgery. The rubber pile bander had just come into fashion in the US but the British would have none of it. It was clear that what the bander did could be bettered by conventional injections and the rest could be done by standard haemorrhoidectomy. I remember an incident when at the precise moment that Prof. Thompson was doing an abdominoperineal resection seated on a stool between the patient's legs, peering into the cavity through his half-moon glasses, a spurt of blood from a large vessel hit his glasses and face. With the spontaneity of a rehearsed comedy, he turned to me and said, 'Udwadia, please request them not to put the lights off when I am operating.' On cue, I removed his glasses, wiped off the blood and replaced them. 'Ahh! We have the lights again,' he quipped and continued. It doesn't hurt to have a sense of humour while operating.

Gradually, my overseas sabbaticals began getting replaced with Indian and international conferences, and these became new ways to update my skill sets and training. But I soon realized the inadequacy of holding workshops for laparoscopic training and was looking for a more permanent method.

In 2005, Mrs Sybill Storz—chairperson of Karl Storz—requested me to meet her in Delhi. Storz Tuttlingen and the Government of Germany were setting up a joint public-private enterprise for evaluating and promoting maternal care in the north-east of India where maternal mortality was the highest. This was a vast undertaking over three years. Though I am not a gynaecologist, Mrs Storz felt that I should be involved in the project. At the end of three years, this was considered to be one of the best public-private projects. When I met Mrs Storz next, I asked her how a private company could match the financial input of the government in a purely altruistic project. She replied saying that since she had no shareholders to answer to, she could use her profits for whatever cause she chose. I then asked her if she could set up a training centre in

India for MAS training. She said she would keep it in mind. Europe had a financial crisis in 2009 and 2010. In 2011, she arranged for us to meet at a laparoscopic surgery conference. She said she was ready to set up a training centre in India. She had two conditions: no live animal would ever be used and the centre would be purely academic—no Storz product would be promoted. In response, I put forth two conditions of my own: Dr Ulhas Gadgil—whom I had worked with at the Johnson and Johnson training centre—would be the director and this would be an autonomous training centre run by surgeons for surgeons.

Mrs Storz accepted my terms. There was no paperwork and no documents. One of the finest training centres for MAS in the world was set up with just a handshake. Mrs Storz did nothing in half measures; I was staggered by the quantum of funds pumped into what was a purely altruistic venture. The quality of equipment provided was the best, the quantity, humongous—including the latest HD cameras, 3D laparoscopy equipment, virtual reality and simulator equipment for every speciality including flexible endoscopy. During the eight years I was chairman of ceMAST, we established affiliations with several associations and societies including the Royal College of Surgeons of England and the Society of Endoscopic and Laparoscopic Surgeons of Asia (ELSA). ceMAST trained over 8000 surgeons in fourteen specialities of MAS.

Aware of the vast, unfulfilled demand for training in MAS in India, ceMAST started making forays into distance learning and had started to prepare courses for the disciplines when it was abruptly closed at short notice. Thanks largely to the managerial and negotiation skills of Dr Suchitra Bindoria, ceMAST has risen from the ashes in its new avatar as the Institute of Indian Medical and Minimal Access Surgery Training (IMMAST) performing the same activities, and run through Sun Pharma.

From 1970, the quantum of clinical and surgical work I was doing surpassed my wildest dreams. I was now attached to JJ, Breach Candy, Hinduja, Parsee General, Masina and was a consultant to the armed forces and the central railways. I also held committee positions in national and international surgery associations and found myself increasingly inundated under an avalanche of work. I could weather through the next few decades thanks only to my secretaries Mani Framroze from 1967 up to 1982 when she had to leave because of her young children, followed by Celina D'souza from 1984 till today and Pervin Dhaboora from 1982 till two years ago, when she retired due to health reasons. In addition, Pervin did all the secretarial work for all the associations and the papers and books published during these years. All three of them gave sanity and system to patient care at my clinic, and ensured that I had my sanity, kept my cool and retained my sense of humour. They will always remain invaluable, unforgettable.

Continuing on a personal note, of my several failures, I would consider the management of my own family one of the most significant. My wife Khorshed has a mind of her own and certainly cannot be pushed around by anyone. It was purely her devotion to me and solidarity with my work that permitted me to work from 7.30 a.m. to 10 p.m. and, after dinner, spend time in my study, reading and writing. She staunchly supported my several travels to rural India for the cause of laparoscopy. I would try to compensate by taking Khorshed to every conference with me—and there were several—so we travelled all over India and the world together but there were several weeks in a row that she spent with housework, playing the piano, teaching the children and waiting for me.

I tried to keep Sunday for the family, especially the children, but there was also competition with golf. We took motoring holidays in India and in Europe, punctuated with daily arguments on who would drive. Although I was a middle-rank student throughout my school and college life, I always expected the children to do better than me. This, I am sure, is an ego problem with most parents where we would compare our children's performance with that of the children of our friends. I am now convinced that doing well in school or college has nothing to do with one's performance in life. If I were to live my life all over again, there are two things I would change drastically: I would never harass the children for being middle-of-the-road students and I would have taken far more holidays with Khorshed and the children.

Surgeons of my period are blessed to have worked and coped with changes during the time of fantastic, unprecedented growth in surgery. However, we cannot be foolish enough to be smug. It is my belief that at the rate at which surgical progress will zoom over the next ten years, it will see advances equal to, if not surpassing, what we have seen in the last seventy years!

MAS is just the beginning. Surgery will get smaller and safer but the smaller will become incomprehensibly bizarre. Mini-robots, the size of an atom, could engineer intracorporeal changes in nanos, much smaller than the size of an atom, to make the nanos carry out intracorporeal manoeuvres like target delivery for drugs to eliminate disease cells as in cancer. Today's surgeons will see a future that could be wilder than the craziest of science-fiction stories. My ultimate surgeon of all time is John Hunter, the eighteenth-century surgeon.

I wholeheartedly concur with his prediction that, 'Surgery, gaining much from the general advancement of knowledge (note knowledge, not surgery) will be rendered both knifeless and bloodless.' The future of surgery will always remain an exciting, life-giving enigma that knows no end.

14

My Ultimate Mentor

My father was, is and will always be my ultimate mentor, both as a doctor and even more so as a human being. He was not a surgeon but had he been one, he would have been first-rate. I am happy and proud that he was a wonderful GP, a family physician who was part of the family of every patient he treated.

Born in 1898, Erach Rustomji Udwadia was the youngest of three sons of Rustomji Edalji Udwadia and Meherbai. His eldest brother Ratansha went off to China at a very young age to try and make his fortune. Because of a neurological problem, his other brother had difficulty walking and in making synchronized movements and so, he couldn't work.

From an early age, Daddy wanted to be a doctor. He did his pre-medical at Wilson College, joined Grant Medical

College (GMC) in 1917 and graduated in 1922. He was a good sportsman and was in the GMC's Cricket XI for all five years and captained it in his final year.

There weren't many colleges in Bombay in the early 1920s and most of the top college cricketers were either in St Xavier's or Elphinstone. And almost invariably, one of these two won the intercollegiate cricket trophy. But the year my father was Grant's cricket captain, GMC won the trophy. This was the first time this had happened and there was jubilation in the college. The day after the tournament's finals, my father was summoned by Grant's dean Major B. Higham. He went to the dean's office, expecting to be congratulated.

'Udwadia,' Higham told him, 'you played an excellent innings, but I am very disappointed with you.' My father, who was walking on air, came down to earth with a thud. 'When you were given out leg-before-wicket,' the dean went on, 'you stood your ground for a few seconds. Cricket is a gentleman's game and the moment you are declared out, you must walk. The umpire is not to be questioned.' The lines of correct behaviour were drawn clear and sharp in 1922! However, one of my treasured possessions is a copy of a testimonial given by Major Higham to my father dated 1922, appreciating his scholastic, sporting and personal qualities.

Wanting to become a surgeon, my father joined Masina Hospital, the first private hospital in Bombay. But when my grandfather, a mill weaving master, retired without a pension or savings, Daddy had to support the family and consequently became a GP.

Daddy's first dispensary was in the heart of Bombay's mill district. He later set up another one in Dongri, also in a poor area. Once he felt he was well-settled, he married. My mother

Perin and he had four sons—Farokh, myself, Darius and Firdaus.

I was blessed to have a very close relationship with my father. As a medical student, after cricket practice at GS College Stadium in Parel, I would stroll over to watch Daddy at work. Even after I returned from the UK with an FRCS and was struggling to build my private practice, I would often land up at his dispensary. I learnt as much—if not more—there, as I did at KEM.

Daddy had two assistants, Dr Rustomji Mirza and Mr Farro, a compounder. Most of his patients were poor and suffered from tuberculosis (TB). But even though he was fully aware of how infectious TB was, he'd ask them to sit near him. I pleaded with him to wear a mask, but he refused. He could not talk freely through a mask, he said. Moreover, he did not want his patients to feel that their doctor was frightened of treating them. He never hurried a patient, even if the waiting room was packed. He used to say that he had only one patient—the one he was talking to.

Once, when a TB patient came to Daddy, Dr Mirza pointed out that he hadn't paid his fees for three months. 'Rustomji,' my father said, 'give him his streptomycin and a B-complex injection.' When Dr Mirza and the patient went to the treatment room for the injections, Daddy pulled out the fat register of pending accounts, drew bold lines across three pages of the patient's dues, and wrote 'Paid in full'. On Dr Mirza's return to the consulting room, Daddy pretended to be annoyed and told him, 'You're wrong, Rustomji. This man paid me a few days ago.' Dr Mirza opened the register and saw that all the entries had been cancelled. I'm sure he knew what Daddy had been up to!

I recall another incident that has always stayed with me. One monsoon night around 10 p.m., after Daddy and I had locked up the dispensary and were sitting in our small Morris Minor, drenched from the rain, all ready to leave for home, I saw a man in a blanket that was shielding him from the pelting rain walking towards the dispensary. Fortunately, Daddy had not seen him and I hoped we could get away. Unfortunately, the car didn't start right away, but when it did and Daddy switched on the headlights, he saw the man standing near the dispensary's entrance.

'He must be a patient,' Daddy said.

'Maybe,' I told him, 'but it's late. You can see him tomorrow.'

'No,' my father said. 'If he has come so late, he obviously needs to see me.'

So, we got out and took the man up to the dispensary, where my father examined him and gave him medication.

I'll never forget one night visit I made with Daddy. A man showed up at our door around 1.30 a.m. and said his wife was very ill and that he wanted Pitaji—that's what many patients called Daddy—to examine her. When I woke Daddy up, he asked me if I'd like to accompany him. It was two months before my final MBBS exam and I'd been studying, but I said yes, and the three of us drove to the patient. Whenever Daddy made a home visit, he carried a large metal box which opened like a three-layered concertina and had all kinds of medications in it. We climbed three flights of rickety stairs and entered a dimly-lit room with about fifteen people sitting or sleeping on the floor. On a mattress in the middle of the room was an obese lady, gasping for breath.

After he'd examined her, Daddy said that she required intravenous deriphyllin. He squatted on the ground, loaded the syringe, but couldn't locate her vein. I told him it was going to be very difficult finding a vein in such poor light. 'We must try,' he replied. Then he got on to his knees and tried again. It took him two tries, but he was finally able to slowly inject the drug into her.

After fifteen minutes, the lady's breathing improved, but we waited another twenty minutes to make sure that she was doing well. As we rose to go, the patient's husband asked Daddy what his fees were. 'Three rupees,' Daddy replied without a moment's hesitation. The husband put his hand in his shirt pocket and took out some one-rupee notes. Making sure that everyone was watching him, the man handed Daddy three.

The fee that Daddy had charged bothered me, but I kept quiet until we were on the way home.

'Daddy,' I told my father, 'you spent more than two hours there—squatting, kneeling, hunting for the vein, and waiting for the drug to take effect. Why did you charge only three rupees?'

'Did you see how many people were in that small room?' Daddy asked me angrily. 'Some of them had probably not even eaten that evening. How much did you want me to charge— twenty rupees, thirty rupees?'

'If you thought they were so poor, why did you charge anything at all?' I shot back.

Daddy was silent for a few seconds. Then he said, 'The poor have a far greater sense of self-respect and dignity than the rich. If I had said no fees in front of all those people, the husband would have felt offended. He did not want my charity, he wanted to pay me whatever I asked. He was able to maintain his respect.'

We lived in a quiet lane with other middle- and upper-middle-class families of different faiths. Four houses down from ours lived a young girl with TB meningitis. Every morning, before patients came to see him at home, my father would visit her. Those were the days before streptomycin; there was nothing Daddy could do for her—he saw her only because he cared.

One morning, Daddy came home with tears in his eyes. She had passed away.

'Quickly,' Daddy told us, 'before your school bus comes, go over and say your prayers near her.'

Whenever Daddy came home from work, the whole house lit up. He always had something interesting to say, something to laugh about. And although, by the time he returned, Farokh and I would have had our dinner, he would call us and put the best piece of mutton or fish from his plate into our mouths. Whenever Mummy complained to him about how mischievous we'd been, he'd put on a stern face and give us a scolding. But his eyes were smiling and we knew he was doing it only to appease her.

On the very rare occasions when Daddy became angry with us, he would shout, 'Bustarny, you stupid Bustarny, this is a stupid Bustarny thing to do.' That was the limit of his cussing. We brothers never found the meaning of the word Daddy had made up: 'Bustarny!'

I learnt from my father that a patient is not a case but a human being who needs help. He taught me that kindness and empathy were as vital as the treatment, in fact, often more so. From him, I learnt that it is more important, more difficult and more meaningful to take care of the poor than the well-to-do.

One of Daddy's favourite stories was about Ambroise Paré, the French surgeon who whittled the ego of surgeons when he wrote, 'I dressed the wound, but God healed him.'* Pare was the royal surgeon to five monarchs of France, including Louis XIV, the Sun King. On one occasion, he kept his royal patient waiting for over two hours. He sheepishly entered the royal chamber, eyes downcast, to face a raging monarch, 'You have kept me waiting! You will treat your monarch better than your patients!' Eyes still downcast, Paré replied, 'I cannot, my Lord, I cannot.' In an incredulous voice, Louis XIV demanded, 'Why can you not treat your king better than your patients?' Paré raised his eyes to meet the King's and said, 'Because sire, I treat all my patients as kings and queens.'

My father kept working until the day he was admitted to hospital with chest pain. He passed away the next morning. He was eighty-six. That afternoon, many people from the mill area came to the Tower of Silence and told us that hundreds more had wanted to come too. The Shiv Sena asked every shop in the vicinity of Daddy's dispensary to down their shutters during Daddy's funeral as a gesture of respect.

My father was and is my idol, my hero and my mentor. My medical-college professors taught me the science of surgery. Through the life he lived, my father taught me humility and compassion, the art of medicine, what it means and takes to be a good doctor. Even today, whenever I face a problem, I turn to him and ask what he would do if he were in my place. He always has an answer for me.

---

* Uh.edu.

Acknowledgements

More than Just Surgery would not have been possible without:

My family—Khorshed, Rushad, Dinaz, Ashad—without whose dedicated love and support little would be possible and nothing would be worthwhile.

My father and all my numerous mentors—whether mentioned or not in the book—who moulded and made me, cleared the path and showed me the way.

My teachers—colleagues, peers, residents and students from whom I learnt more than I taught. And the nurses and technicians who have given me knowledge and vision over the decades.

My patients—each one I have looked after over 67 years has been a gift that has paved the road in my journey towards becoming a better surgeon.

Gayatri Pahlajani, who has been on this project almost from its inception. She has been a counsellor and friend, quietened my tantrums and has edited the thousands of words written by me for each chapter (to my regret!), to a form and volume acceptable to the publisher, yet keeping the gist intact. We have had our rows and differences, defused by her cool, happy, humorous ability of combining conflicting views, and making the collaboration stronger.

Titoo Ahluwalia, friend and buddy of over 40 years, who is bubblier than champagne, is the guiding angel of all boy scouts, is ever ready to help, and is a specialist in the restoration of floundering causes. He has worked on this book in several diverse aspects with greater enthusiasm, passion, energy, thought and joy than I have! He is one of a kind, unique in every way.

Ashok Mahadevan, brought in towards the completion of the book by Titoo to give the ultimate quality of his quick expert editorship of all chapters, which he carried out graciously, rapidly and with his customary perfection.

Gurveen Chadha, senior commissioning editor, in charge of this book on behalf of Penguin Random House. She completely changed my preconception of publishers. Over a year I have found her kind, willing to help in every way, making graceful allowances for my ignorance of the entire process and accepting reasons for my delay with compassion. I acknowledge with thanks the support of Ralph Rebello and the Penguin Random House staff from the various teams.

Lastly, I'd also like to thank Vaishali Suresh Parab, who has read and printed reams and reams of my illegible writing, copied hours of dictation, corrected and recorrected every page of my literary and verbal diarrhoea till the present form, pleasantly, without any complaint, as promptly as possible.